The Fast, F

How to Eat, Fast
& Live Longer

Dr. Paul Cronin

Disclaimer & Privacy Policy:

ISBN: 9781973187226
Published by PACC Ltd

Index

Introduction

I must start this book with two apologies. The first is to Dr Michael Mosley who did a BBC Horizon documentary from which I stole the subtitle of this book. It was an excellent documentary and you should check it out sometime.

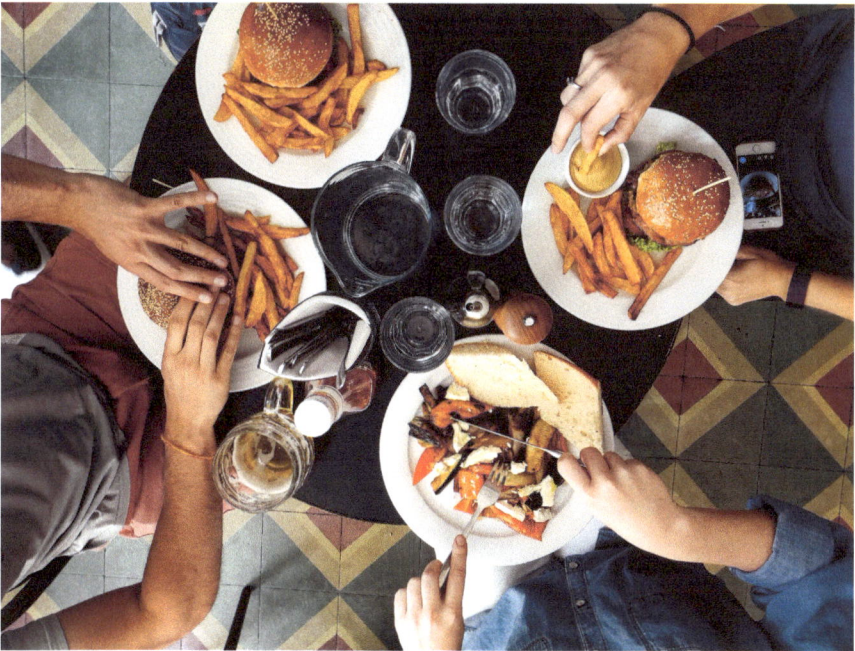

The second apology is to you too, dear reader, or at least the possibly less observant ones. Anyone who misread the title and thought this was a guide to eating fast food and living longer and failed to notice the comma. The comma may seem small and inconsequential but it is vital as you shall see.

A little bit about you

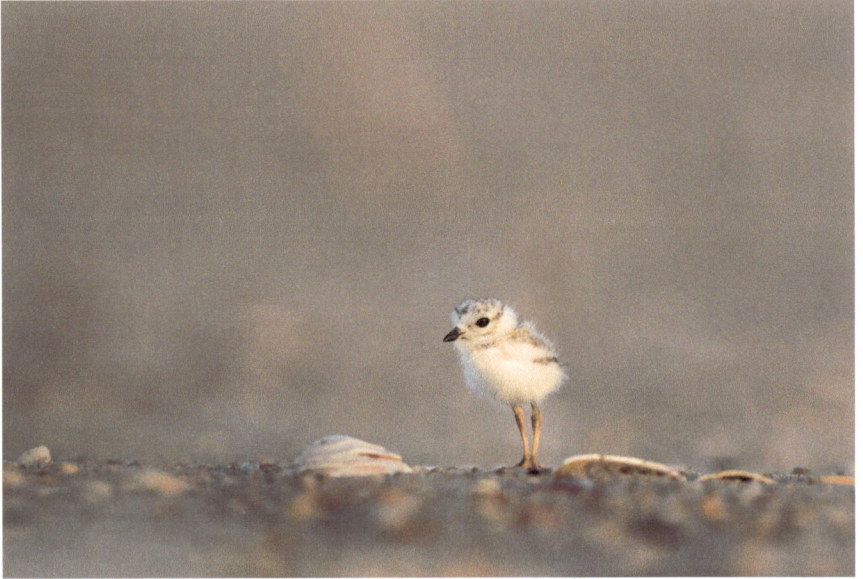

I suspect that if you have taken a look at this book you have, or have had, problems with weight gain either now or in the past. You may have tried various diets and found them wanting. You might have been recommended to read this by a friend or work colleague. Hopefully, someone who has already read it and found it useful.

This is a book about diet and lifestyle and it will help with weight problems, but it is also mostly about health and longevity. Living longer and fitter and hopefully a little happier too.

You might feel a little lost and confused amidst the wealth of conflicting advice out there about what to eat and what to do. There is conflicting advice and it is easy to see why.

An old medical school joke was that if you had ten doctors in a room you could probably get twenty different opinions. We don't always agree with each other, even if we are looking at exactly the same data.

So what is this book aiming to do?

Well, hopefully, it will give you some new information. It will have new stuff but it will also repeat some stuff I know you already know. I do hope it will inspire you to try out some of the more radical ideas and see if they work for you. Nothing works for everyone but everything is worth trying until you find the one thing that works best for you.

I also hope you enjoy reading it as much as I have enjoyed writing it.

A little bit about me

I qualified in medicine at Manchester University in 1985. I was a full-time GP for 14 years, I gradually sidestepped into cosmetic medicine and now anti-ageing medicine. The human body has always held a fascination for me. At the age of seven, I declared I wanted to be a doctor. Even then, as a child, I moulded plasticine heads and carved delicate facial features on them. I now have the immense privilege of sculpting the human form when I perform liposuction and facial treatments. It is a truly amazing thing to see the smiles on the patients when they come back for their review appointments.

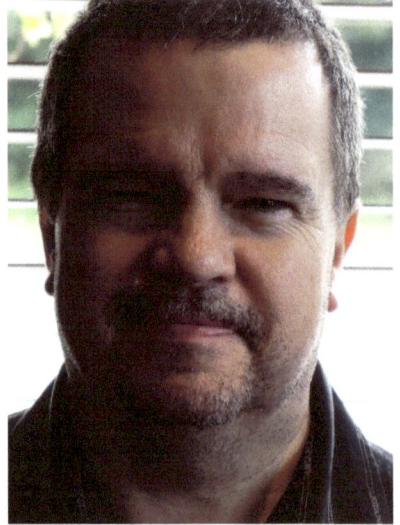

Personally, I have had a significant weight problem for most of my life (way too fond of chocolate). More recently I developed high blood pressure. (I am now 55 so I wasn't really shocked). But when I was struggling to control the readings despite two different anti-hypertensives and having to consider adding a third I thought there must be something better than this.

At about that time I saw Michael Mosley's documentary and was introduced to the concept of alternate day fasting. I had tried most diets over the years and had been fairly successful with the low carb or Atkins approach, but what interested me most about the alternate day fasting concept is that it was not really about losing weight it was more about controlling blood pressure and improving diabetes and cholesterol. It was mainly aimed at improving longevity. So anything was worth a go.

Well, I thrust into the diet with my usual relish, (you'll have to forgive the foody puns) and found that I was able to quickly lose over a stone in weight whilst not really having to feel very hungry and more importantly not having to totally exclude any foods from my diet.

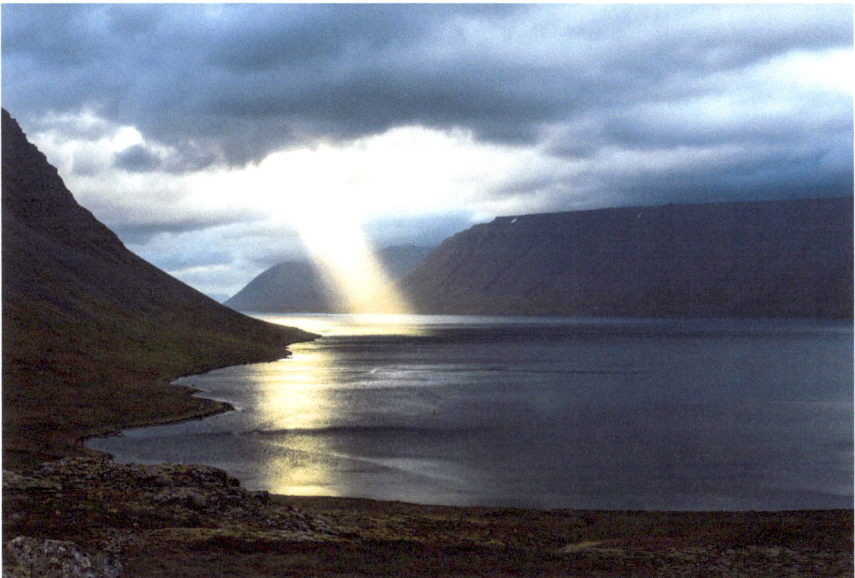

Most importantly I am now able to report that my blood pressure is better controlled now without any medication than it was on two separate drugs before the weight loss.

So I am certainly happy that I found this solution and it gels well with a whole lot of other information I have been gathering over the years about diet, exercise, lifestyle, and even spiritual wellness.

So having explained a little bit about me let me tell you a bit about this book.

I will purposely keep it short, sweet and simple. For two reasons. Firstly I want it to be easy to read so you will get through it quickly and get started on implementing the suggestions. Secondly, I profess no major inclination to literary prowess, (wow those are big words for me) so I could probably not make it too verbose even if I tried.

More importantly, I want this simple little book to inform and inspire you to perhaps do your own research into this field and make your own mind up about what works for you. I was fed up with the one size fits all philosophy of many diets and nutritional "gurus". Human beings are very different individuals and one reason there are so many different opinions is that all things cannot work for all people. You have to find your own solution which works for you. I hope this book provides you with a new and interesting insight into some of the possible strategies which will help you to peak health and a long, happy and fulfilled life.

We are all inevitably going to die. I don't want or intend to live forever. I don't want to live to 110 if I spend the last 20 years drooling from my mouth in a nursing home. I would be very happy to die at 95 if at 94 I was white-river rafting down the Grand Canyon.

This is not about duration. It is about quality.

I want to be as healthy as I can be right up until the moment I die.

You are what you eat

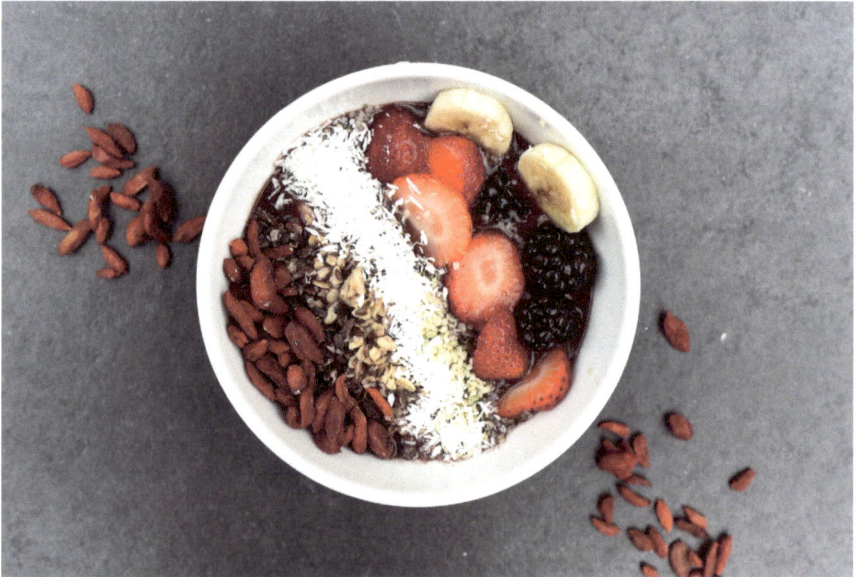

This term has been overused by so many people that I didn't really want to use it. But the simple fact is that it is true. If you think about it is is entirely obvious. Your body is in a constant state of change. It is in a constant state of repair. Your stomach lining cells last only a few days, skin cells only last a few weeks, red blood cells can survive a few months, bone cells can last for many years and it is believed that most of the cells in your brain last a lifetime, hopefully.

This high turnover of many of the cells and tissues drives a constant demand for fuel and protein to rebuild them. Human beings are fairly inefficient in terms of calorific efficiency.

Quite a lot of the energy we consume is wasted in the mechanism of turning food into body parts.

One of the biggest problems is making sure that we have the right ingredients at the right time. If you have a recipe for a chocolate cake (can you see the theme here?) it has to have exactly the right amounts of flour, sugar, cocoa and eggs. Too much of any one ingredient spoils the cake.

One obvious problem with this is that depending on what we're trying to make (body parts, not cakes) the food we eat at that time may not have exactly the right proportions of in-gredients we need. So we need stores of stuff.

The main thing we need to store is fuel and the main fuel we use is sugar. Sugar is in fact stored in two forms in the body. It is stored in the liver as glycogen and in the tissues as fat. The main fat that most people are aware of is subcutaneous fat. Fat just under the skin. But there are many deposits of fat throughout the body some more visible than others. From a health and longevity point of view, the most important store of fat is intra-abdominal fat. Fat stored within the abdominal cavity. This is a major marker for many disease processes and is also a cause of occasional concern for liposuction surgeons. This fat which is inside the body rather than just under the skin is not available for removal with a liposuction cannula and this can cause problems for the patient when the shape improvement is not as much as they want be-cause this fat is not reachable.

There are ways to get rid of this fat which we will discover later but suffice it to say that all fat wherever it is stored is the body's main long term fuel storage.

Vitamins and minerals are stored in a variety of sites around the body, calcium in the bones for example and we only need access to these in fairly small quantities but many are still vital to a healthy life and more importantly a healthy lifespan.

Protein is a funny one as we don't really store it anywhere as such but it is 'recyclable' sort of, in that we can take protein from an area considered less important and give it to another considered more important. An extreme example of this is seen in pregnancy when even if the mother is suffering from malnutrition she will leach protein from her own muscles to provide the baby with its growing needs.

We still do require a reasonable supply of easily assimilable protein to replenish that lost through wear and tear.
So with all this turnover we do need a reasonable amount of fuel calories and protein building blocks in our daily diet to replace all the lost tissues and cells.

The most important thing is the balance of all the different types of food. I am personally a firm believer in 'Rainbow food'. This is the concept of making sure that we eat a large variety of different coloured foods. I think the colours are less important than the variety of foodstuffs consumed. Although some recent research has suggested that the colours them-selves may be the beneficial bit. Man should not live on pasta alone, or bread alone, or pretty much anything alone.

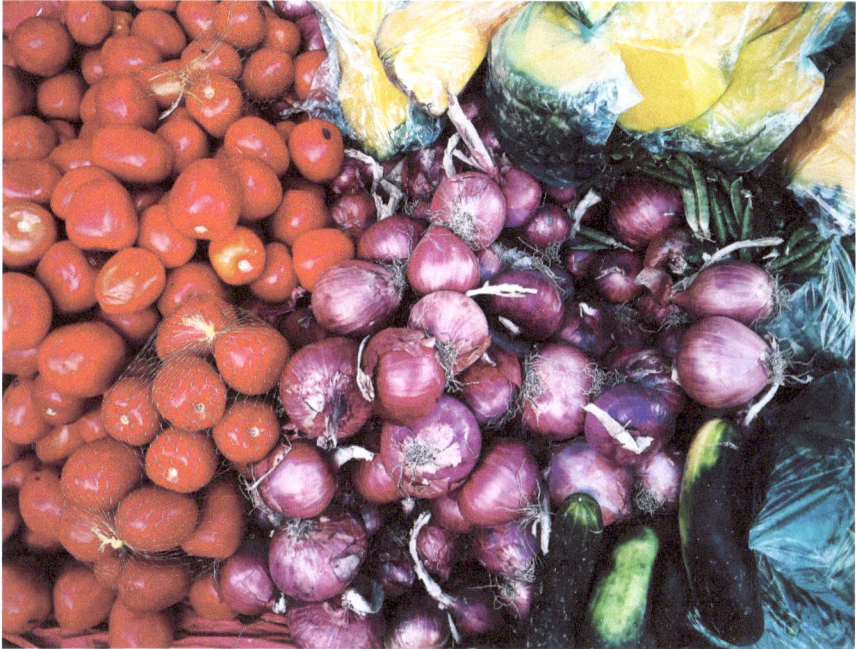

In fact, despite my keenness for the low carb approach there is a well-documented phenomenon sometimes referred to as rabbit starvation, which was common amongst Canadian trappers who in the winter months would feed exclusively on lean protein from rabbit meat and it caused a lot of problems some of which were fatal. Interestingly some research has indicated that it wasn't so much an excess of protein but a reduction or loss of fat which provoked the symptoms. On a similar vein, the Inuit people of Northern Canada traditionally had a diet of almost exclusively fat and protein.

All food is either carbohydrate, protein or fat. There is nothing else. Anything we can take into our bodies and assimilate in some way is one of these types. Most foods actually contain all of these types to varying degrees.

So whilst meat is primarily a protein it contains a variable amount of fat and a small amount of carbohydrate. Vegetables whilst primarily carbohydrates can contain a significant amount of protein and usually some fat too.

More interestingly there is only one type of food that you can avoid altogether and it isn't fat. It is carbohydrate.

The traditional Inuit diet was almost exclusively animal fat and protein as there was almost no access to vegetable matter. This diet has changed considerably for the modern day Inuit due to influences from the more 'developed world'. The increase in carbohydrates, sugars and convenience foods in their diet is matched with a similar increase in a whole range of 'western diseases' too. More of that later.

Fat makes you fat

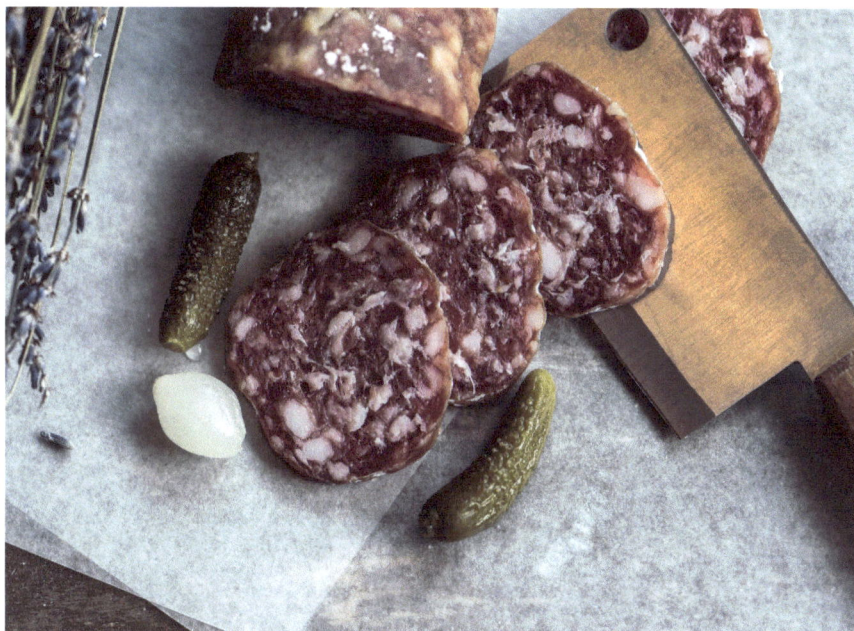

I don't intend to delve deeply into the science here as there is a lot of this information online and plenty has been published in the press. Unfortunately, the establishment got it badly wrong.

Back in the late 50s early 60s the American medical establishment was concerned that Americans where getting too fat. They believed (wrongly) that Americans were eating too much fat. At the time the American diet was roughly 40 to 45 % of daily calories from fat. The American medical establishment decided that it would be better for Americans to eat less fat. (It seems logical I know) So there was an enormous

13

public health campaign to get the population to eat less fat and boy was it successful.

By the early 90s, the percentage of calories from fat in the 'average' American diet had fallen to about 25% Fantastic. Didn't they do well?

However unfortunately over the same time frame, the average weight of the population had gone up.

Americans were getting very much fatter.

So despite a very expensive and high profile public health campaign which had very successfully changed the overall dietary intake in a major way the problem had got worse.

Why?
Fat isn't the problem.
Dietary fat certainly isn't the problem.

In fact, total calories aren't really the problem. The total calories consumed over this time frame had only risen a little.

The population had taken the message on board, hook, line and sinker. The food manufacturers had produced a whole lot of lower fat foods. The stores were full of displays and suggestions on how to lower the fat content of your diet to a 'more healthy' level.

The trouble is if you take something out of a food you have to put something back in its place. The thing they mostly put back in was various forms of carbohydrate.

Next time you are at the supermarket check out the coleslaw. Compare the low-fat version with the 'full fat' version. Try it with the peanut butter.

The ingredients in 'full fat' peanut butter include peanuts and sometimes salt depending on the brand. The ingredients in low-fat peanut butter include a long list of stuff, most of which I have never heard of and some of which I doubt I would even classify as food. In fact, most prepackaged foods at the supermarkets even the ones that don't fall into the low-fat category contain a whole lot of mysterious ingredients designed to improve the flavour or the colour or the shelf life or the 'mouth consistency'. Are these things we really want to be eating? Is guar gum actually food….?

So when the average American managed to reduce his dietary intake of fat he unfortunately also had to increase his dietary intake of carbohydrates. By the way for those of us in the UK the situation was very similar.

Increasing your carbohydrate intake is followed by a necessary increase in your insulin output. Insulin causes your body to store this excess sugar as fat. That is its job. Insulin is a storage hormone.

Unfortunately, long-term increases in carbohydrate consumption go hand in hand with long-term excess insulin production which not only makes you fatter but also deadens the response of your insulin receptors to the action of insulin. Interestingly this increase also deadens your response to leptin another hormone associated with the satiety response.

This is the hormone which is supposed to stop you feeling hungry when you have eaten enough. So as you still feel hungry you continue to stuff carbs into your mouth which then stimulates, even more, insulin and, even more, insulin resistance. This causes your pancreas to work harder at producing, even more, insulin to cope with this increasing insulin resistance.

This all leads to a condition which is now classified as Metabolic Syndrome or Syndrome X or Insulin resistance or Hyperinsulinaemia. Eventually, your pancreas can't cope anymore and you develop type 2 diabetes.

So as well as making Americans very much fatter this strategy also massively increased the incidence of diabetes amongst the American population (and ours too).
So what is the simple yet inevitable answer to this problem? We need to eat less carb.

We probably need to eat more fat too.

Yes, I did say that.

Fat is good.

More later.

The low carb thing

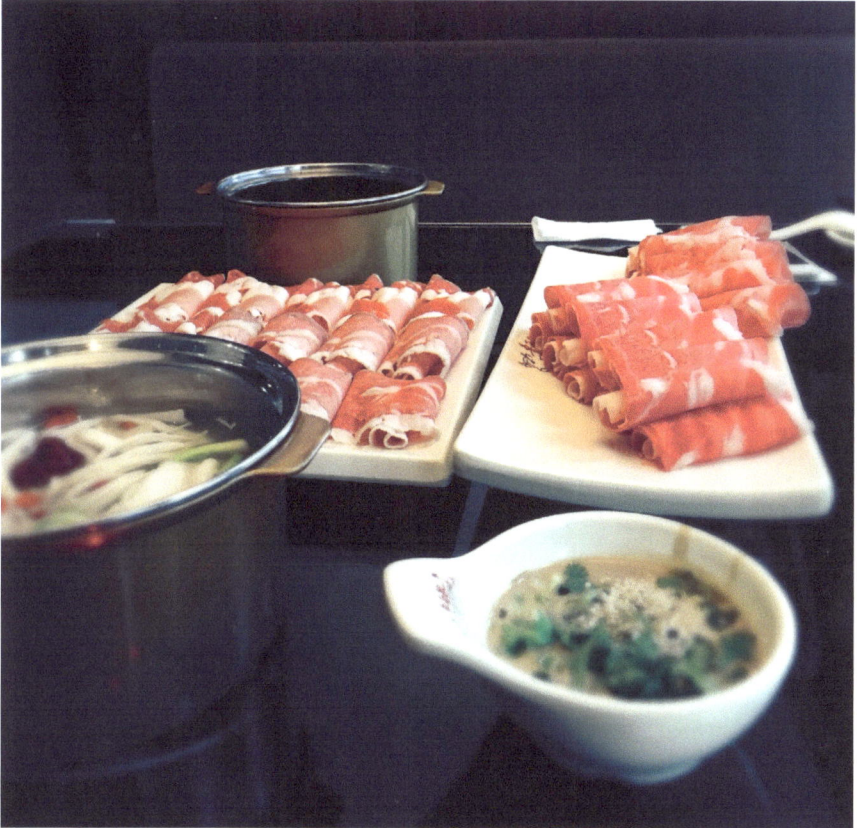

There is no doubt that the low carb diet works. The reasons for this seem obvious after the discussion in the previous chapter. However, this has caused some degree of controversy amongst the medical and dietetic fraternity. I heard an interesting comment on the radio the other day by a 'Nutritional Expert' who was trying to slag off the Atkins diet by saying that it only works by reducing the daily calorie intake.

Big shock.

All diets only work by reducing the calorie intake.

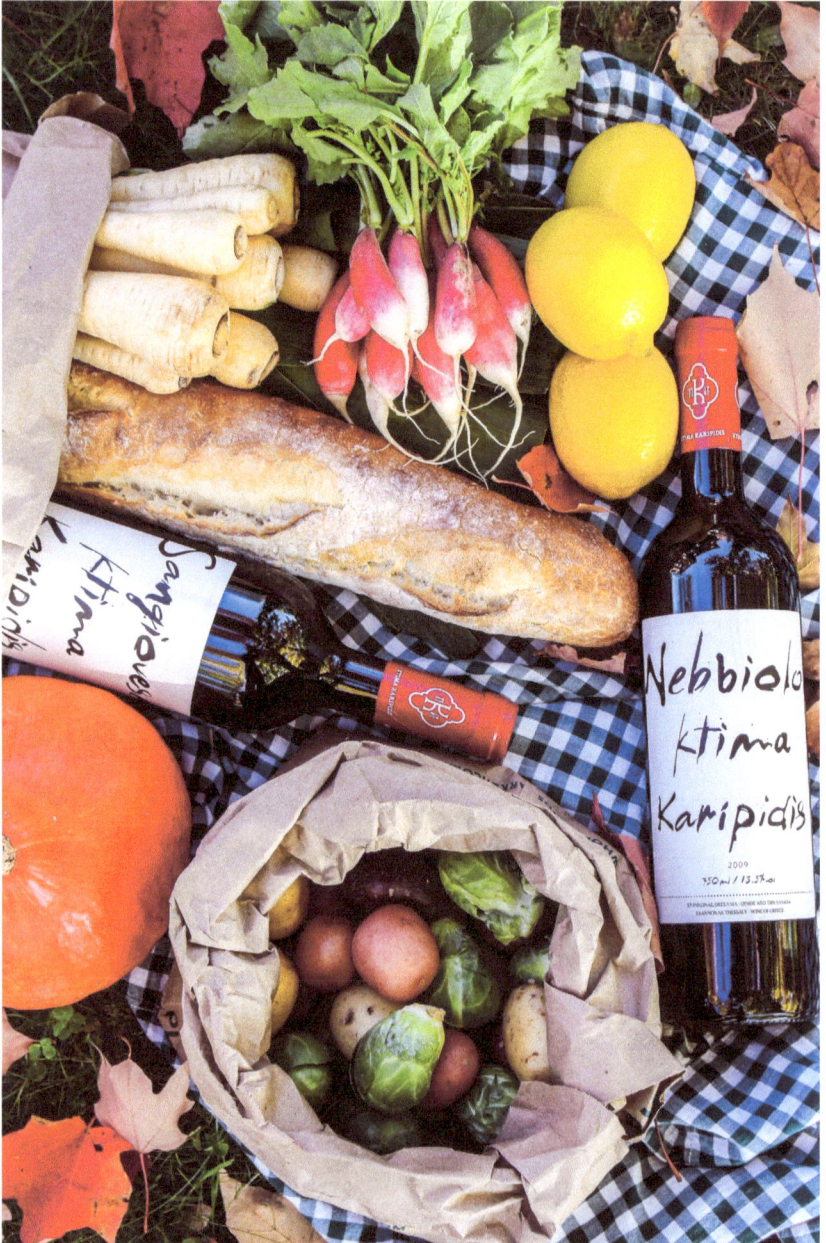

All lifestyle changes which work do so by either increasing the calories burned or reducing the calories consumed, or preferably both.

The only real problem with the low carb approach is a psychological one. Any diet that excludes a significant food or food group will not be something you will do on a long term basis.

Let's get the big DIET word out of the way first.

A DIET is not something you do for a few weeks to lose weight before your summer holiday so you look better in a bikini.

Your DIET is what you eat. It is preferably what you are going to be happy to eat for the rest of your life.

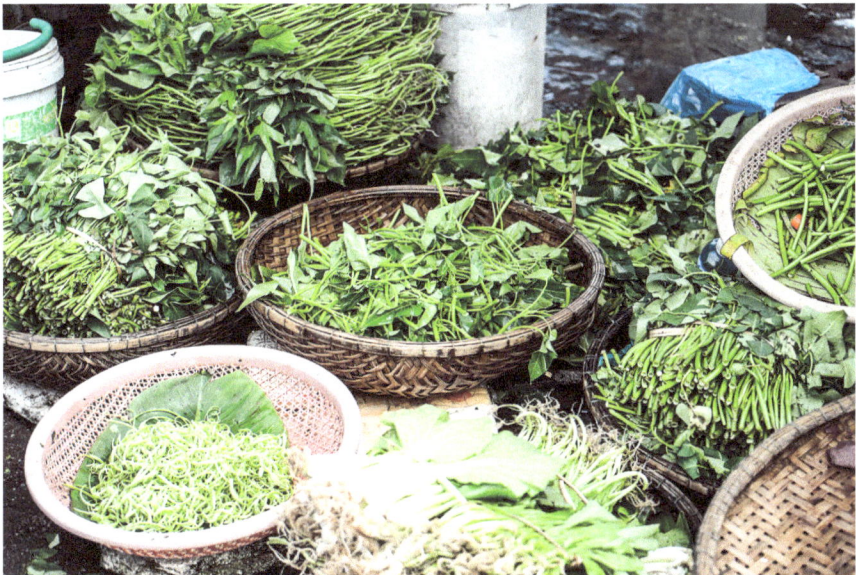

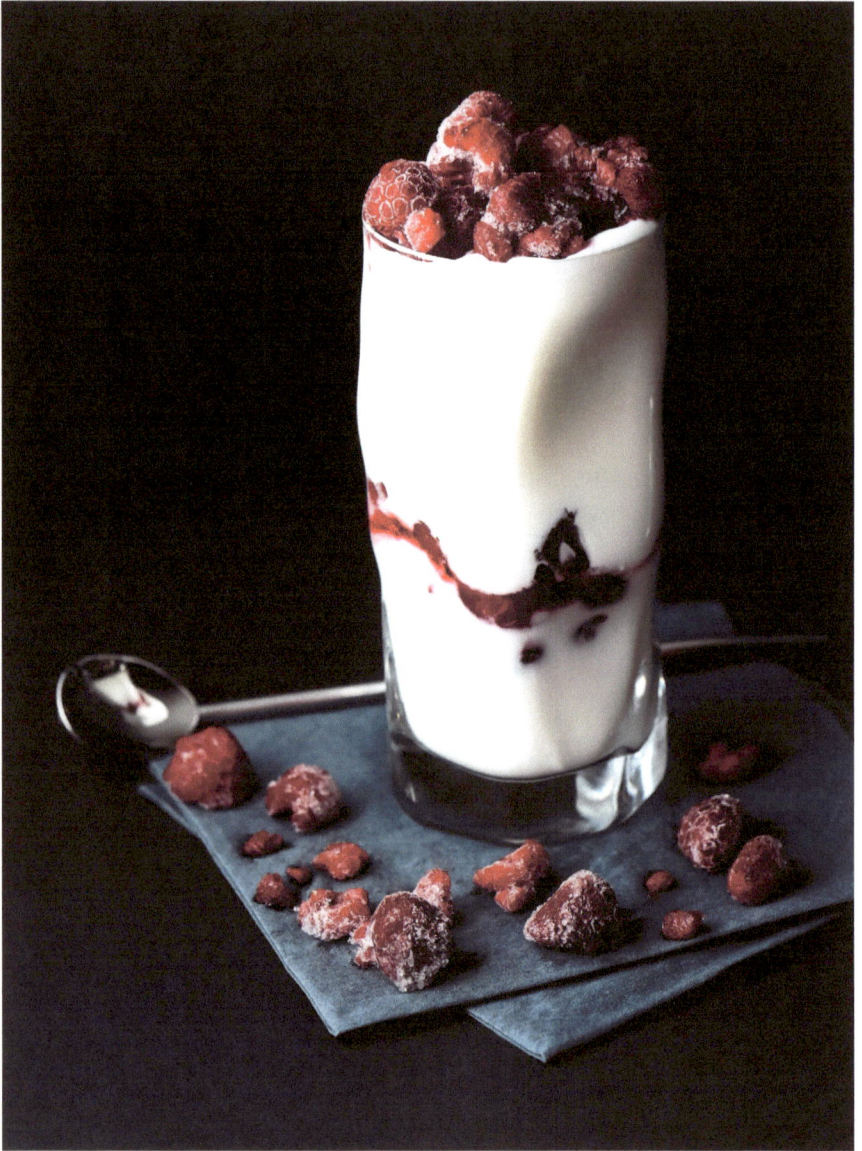

A few months ago I had a patient come to see me for a Vaser Lipo treatment to her tummy and having gone through all the risks etc and explained the recommended diet for the first few weeks after the treatment, she was about to sign the consent form when she asked me.

"When can I go back to my original diet?"

I paused briefly and said "Look down. That is the result of your original diet. If you want to get it back after the treatment then you can go back on your original diet."

I paused again.

"If you don't want it back, then you can never go back to your original diet."

So you need to start to think of your diet as a permanent thing. It needs to be something you will be happy to do forever.

Whilst what you eat is obviously very important. Why you eat is almost more important. If you are reading this because you have a problem with weight then something that you are currently doing is wrong. Something needs to change, something needs to change on a long term basis.

When you were a child your parents probably fretted about how much you ate, as most parents do. If they thought you weren't eating enough then they probably did what most parents do which is to bribe you into eating more.

"If you finish your supper you can have a dessert."

"If you finish that last bit of sausage you can have a piece of chocolate."

This very common practice did often persuade children to eat more of the meat or perhaps taste a new vegetable they weren't interested in. However, it also set up a dangerous precedent.

If you are good we will give you sugar. If you do what you are told you will be rewarded with sweet tasting food. This continues into later life when we reward ourselves with dessert or chocolate to celebrate a success at work or to cheer us up when things have not gone the way we wanted.

Don't get me wrong. Food is good. Tasty food is good. Even fatty food is good(more of this later). It is just too much food which is bad. Too much of any type of food. Too much broccoli is probably bad for you. (Although I suspect too much broccoli would be a hell of a lot…)

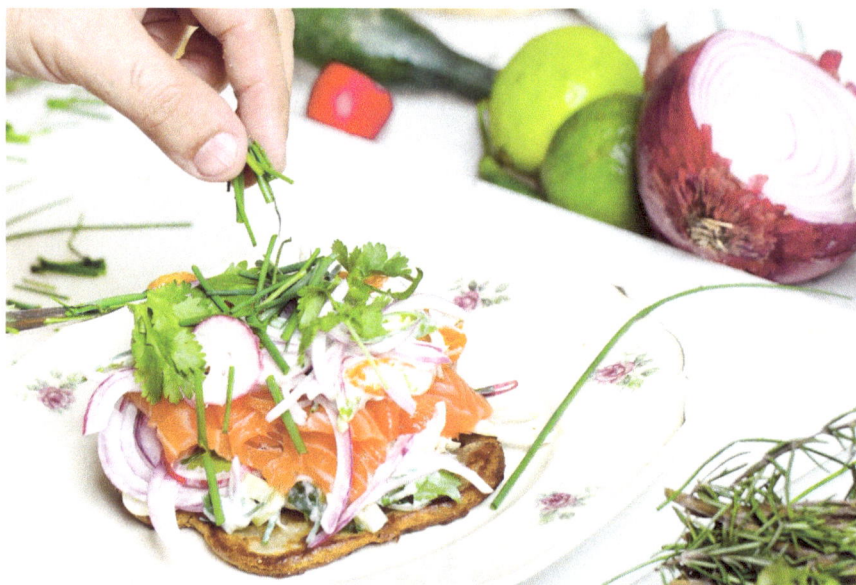

We want to eat because we are hungry. We want to eat because we enjoy the taste. We probably shouldn't eat to cheer ourselves up.

The 'why' is more important than the 'what'. The 'when' is probably pretty important too (again more of that later). Eat if you are hungry. (Although as seen later being hungry isn't going to kill you.) Don't eat more than you need out of habit, or because it is on your plate, or because you paid for it, or because it is lunch time.

Eat to live and live to eat. Just eat less and you'll probably live longer.

Fat is good

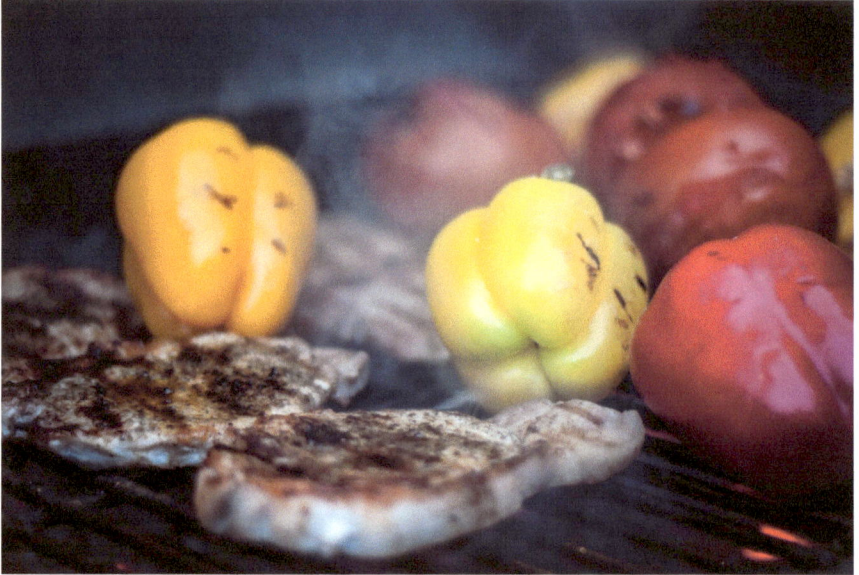

So your diet is something you are going to be prepared to eat forever. It seems that reducing the carb level would be a good idea and whoopee "fat is good"!

Ok, not all fat is good.

Now whilst I hate the overall concept of good foods and bad foods it has to be said that some fats are better than others. As a general rule about all food the more natural and un-touched a product is the better it is likely to be for you. The more processed, the more 'manufactured' it is the less likely it is to be good for you.

Some would even go so far as to advocate eating a very substantial part of your diet as raw food. Food in its freshest most natural state. Preferably just recently plucked from the allotment washed chopped up and eaten.

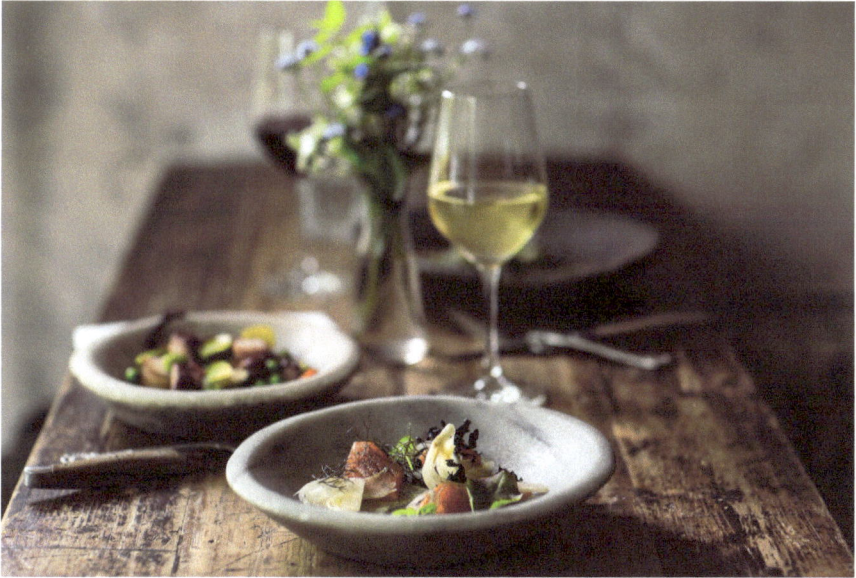

So what percentage of our calories should come from 'good' fats? Can you remember the food pyramid? The triangular diagram which started with cereals at the bottom and ended up with fat and protein at the top. That was all based off sound scientific research, wasn't it?

Unfortunately no. In fact, it was made up by a group associated with funnily enough cereal manufacturers who thought it would be a great way to get you to eat more cereal. It worked, didn't it?

This went hand in hand with the whole thrust of the low fat is good for you diet thingy. We all saw where that got us.

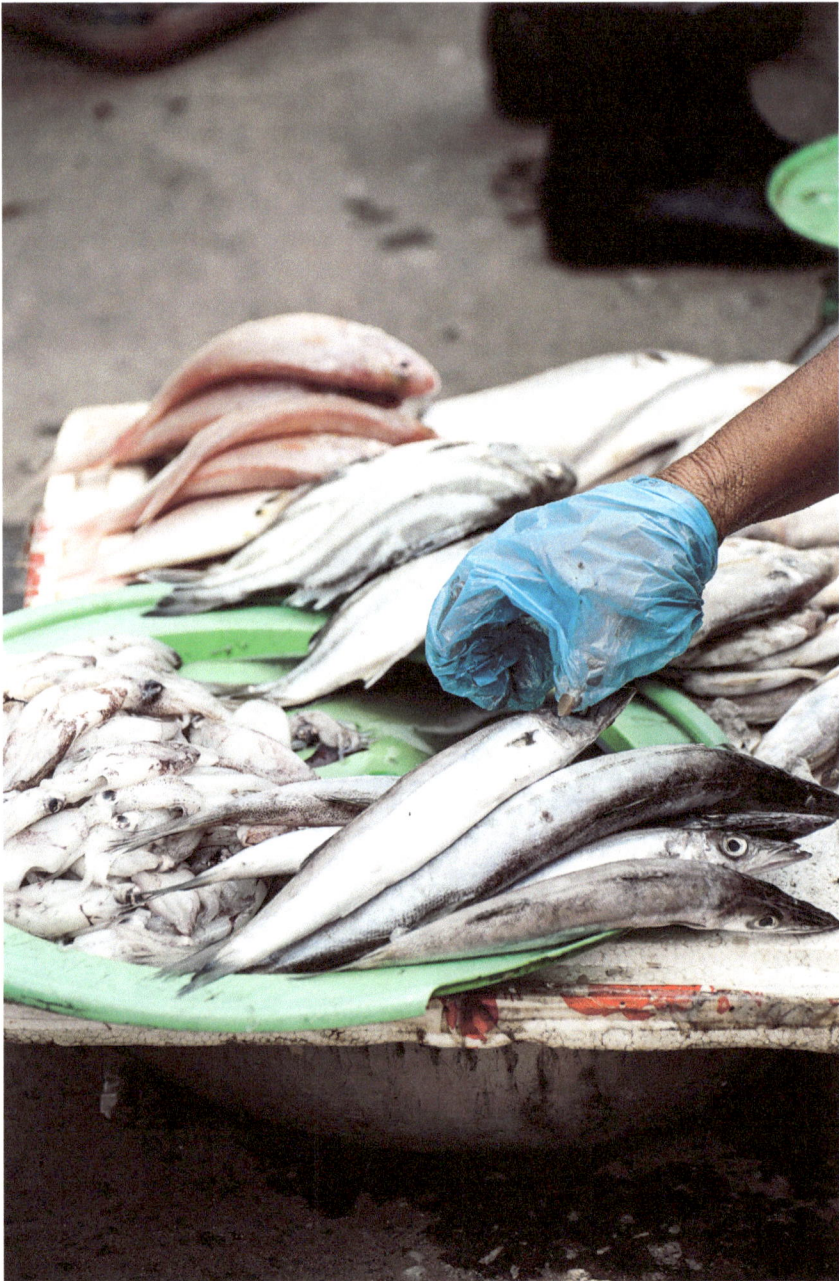

Over the years this has been discussed ad nauseam by various aspects of the medical and health professions. The main contentions being the relative proportions of dietary fat, protein and carb. The vegetarians all wanted to suggest less protein was needed (primarily to reduce our consumption of animals I suspect). The cereal manufacturers and their associates thought we ought to eat more carb and they all, at that time, thought we should eat less fat. This argument has changed only slightly over the years and I don't intend to outline all the details.

Let me simply state my current recommendations to my own patients and let me apologise in advance to any members of the medical profession who might disagree with me. We are each entitled to our own opinions.

My current recommendations to my patients involve the roughly 30/30/40 split that has had various different exponents over the years.

For clarity, my 30/30/40 split is 30% protein 30% carb and 40% "good fats". I know that many of my esteemed colleagues would swap the carb and the fat around but I do think now that the evidence for less carb in the diet is pretty strong.

Notice that I do not advocate a high protein diet. Many people complained about the low carb approach calling it a high protein diet. I prefer to think of the low carb approach as more of a high fat diet but I know that many people don't like the way that sounds in the present climate. Time will tell who is right in this field. Yes, I am arrogant enough to think it will be me…..sorry.

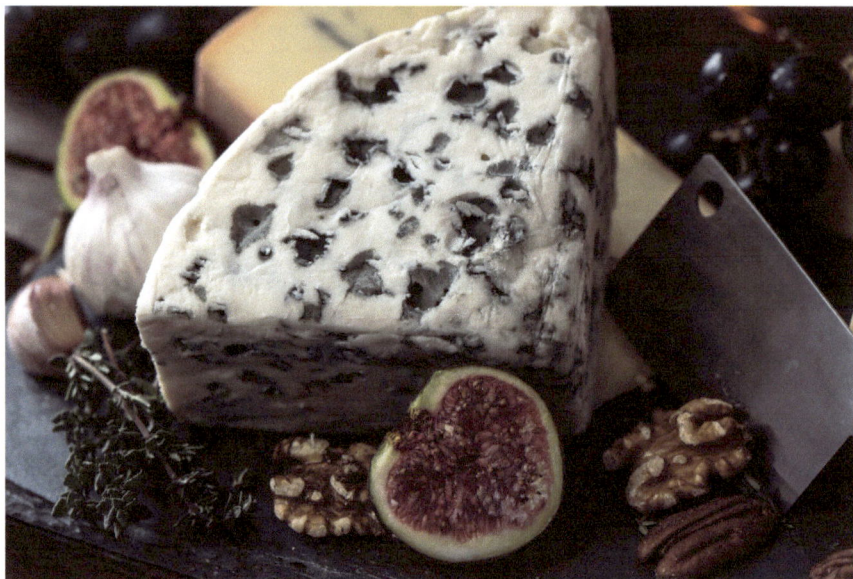

So with regards to fats, which are good and which are bad (or just less good)?

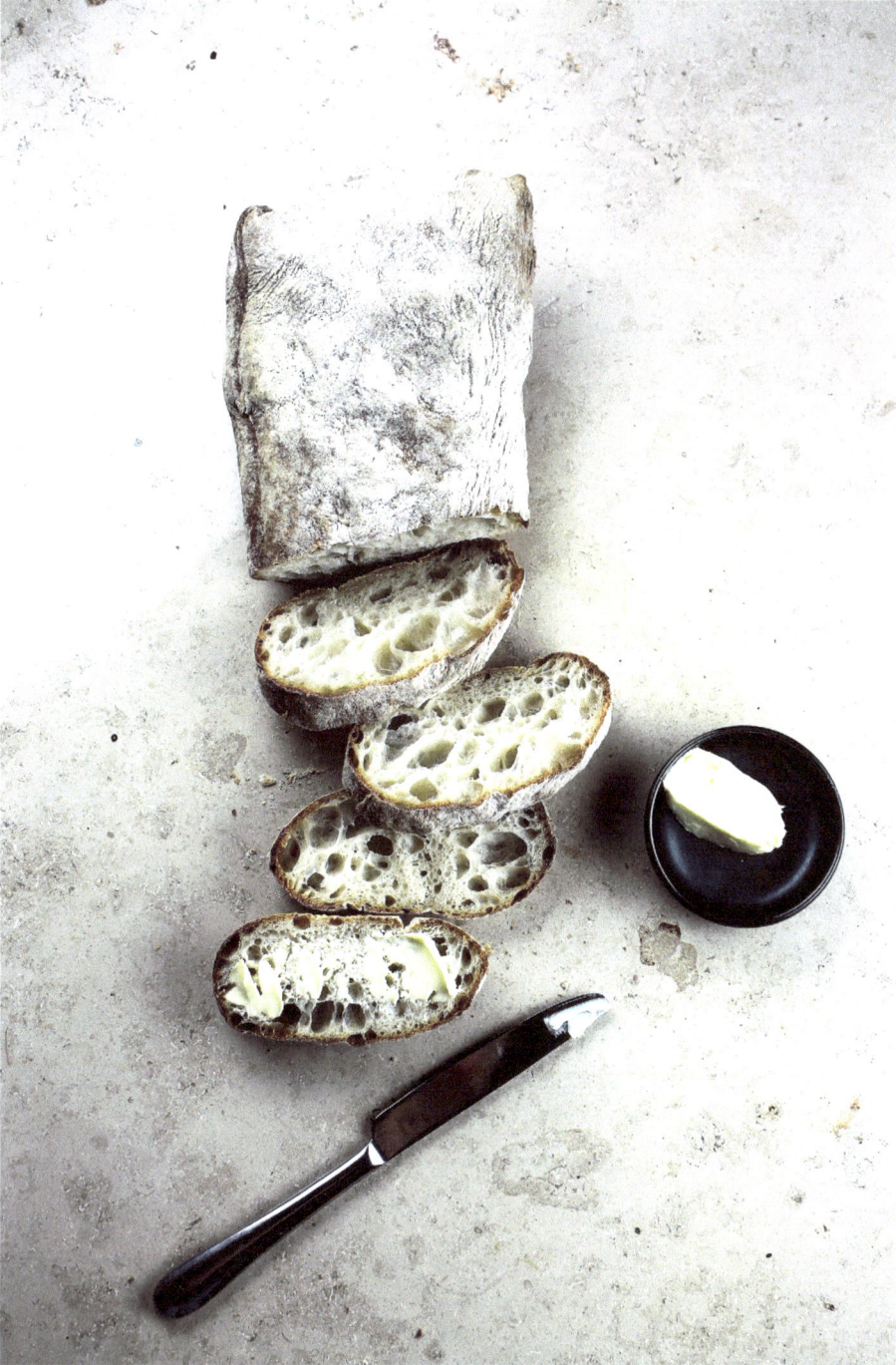

Butter v margarine

Well, to stick with our theme from the previous chapter there is an obvious problem with margarine. If our general trend is to eat more natural food then nothing can be less natural than margarine. Any industry that is known as the yellow fat industry sounds like a none starter to me. But let's look into why this all started.

Yes, we are back in the 50s and 60s again. When the whole idea was to eat less fat the big bugbear was 'saturated fat'. These were perceived as the most heinous of all. Thus manufacturers were persuaded to look for 'healthier' alternatives to saturated fats such as butter etc.

Margarine has been made from various things over the years, at one time it was made from whale blubber. It was invented by a French chemist in 1813 when Emperor Louis Napoleon III offered a prize to anyone who could invent a satisfactory substitute for butter, suitable for use by the armed services and the lower classes.[1]

That makes it sound great, doesn't it?

It originally was made from animal fats but these were substituted with hydrogenated vegetable oils when the whole low-fat thing got going. Now this is where the whole problem

---

[1] ^ *Science Power 9: Atlantic Edition,* McGraw-Hill Ryerson Limited. ISBN 0-07-560905-3.

lies. If you have a liquid vegetable oil and you want to make it into a butter substitute then you have to do various chemical things to it to hydrogenate it to make it thicker and more solid. This hydrogenation process also produces a certain portion of trans fats in the mixture. Suffice it to say that many studies suggest that this form of fat is less than healthy. Also, there is a whole discussion we won't bother to have yet about unsaturated fats and the balance between Omega 3 fatty acids and Omega 6 fatty acids.

Margarine is just one step away from being purely chemical in nature and would go under the category of none foods for me. It gained popularity over the war years due to the scarcity of dairy products and it was able to use the whole low-fat drive to deeply embed itself in the human psyche such that many people especially ladies are so convinced that fat is bad for you that they would never dream of using butter and genuinely 'prefer' to eat margarine.

Can I simply say to these ladies? Margarine is a pretty rough chemical product that has various 'black marks' against it and almost no positives so why not enjoy a small amount of a much better product from a natural source known as butter.

There are many other much better more natural dietary fats such as butter, olive oil, coconut oil etc. Many natural foods such as nuts and oily fish are high in beneficial oils too so really there is no need for margarine whatsoever.

So let's be really clear here.

Please don't eat margarine.

Ever.

Is that clear enough?

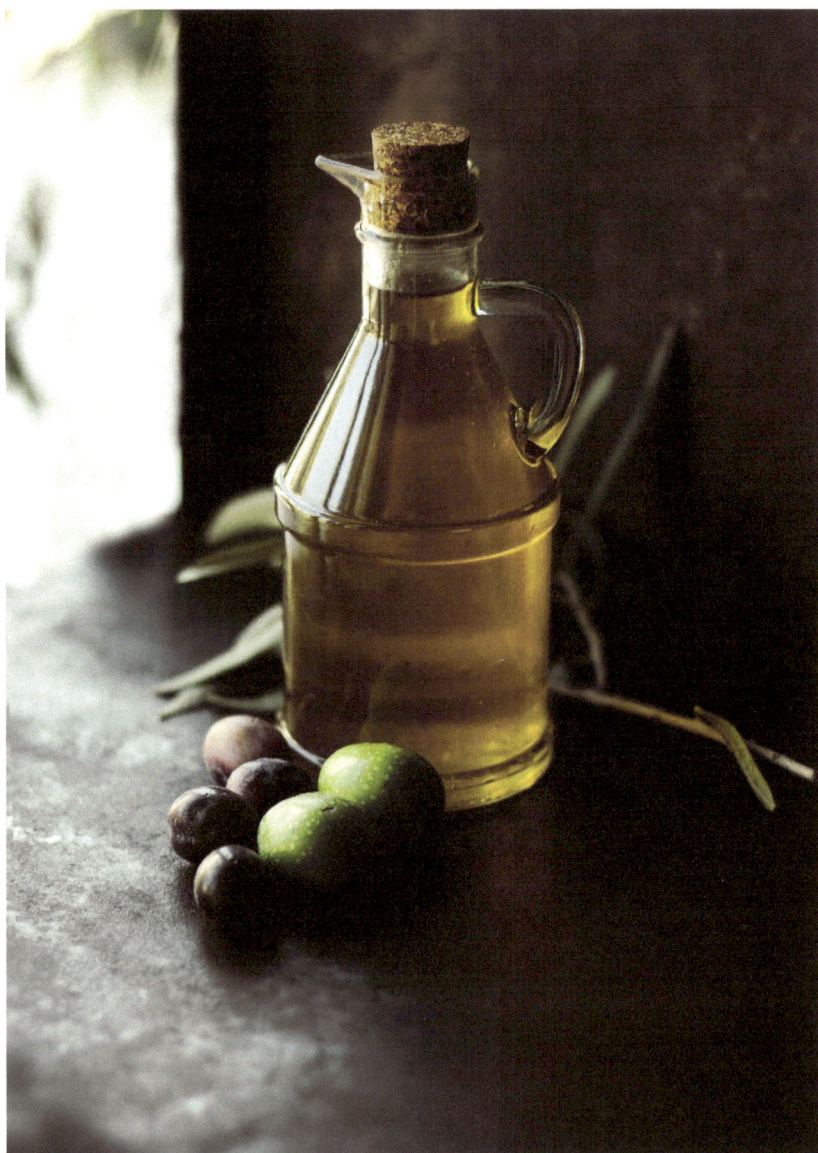

Low-fat foods

While we are on the subject of fat, let's touch again on low-fat foods. By definition, if they've taken the fat out they have had to replace it with something. This is usually carbohydrate or some nonfood stuff such as guar gum and other thickeners. It is simply worth repeating that the best stuff to swallow is usually food in its most basic and unrefined, unprocessed form. Preferably raw.

I tell all my patients to avoid pretty much everything which declares itself as low fat on principle alone. Remember that we said earlier that in fact, we want to eat more 'good fat' and I know some of this 'low fat' rubbish is higher in polyunsaturated fats and vegetable oils but that doesn't necessarily make it any healthier for you. In fact, the current dietary trends in the UK mean that we usually get plenty of omega 6 fatty acids found in vegetable oils etc but not enough omega 3 fatty acids found in marine fish, krill and some nuts etc. So taking onboard a low-fat yoghurt because it is high in polyunsaturated fats may push the balance of 3s to 6s even further.

So when it comes to low fat anything just say no!

Good fats are abundant in fish oils. These are best found in naturally caught fish such as mackerel tuna or wild salmon, but they can be added with appropriate supplementation of cod liver oil or even the latest Krill oil which comes from antarctic regions and is less contaminated with metal toxins. Other good sources of oil include avocados and olive oil.

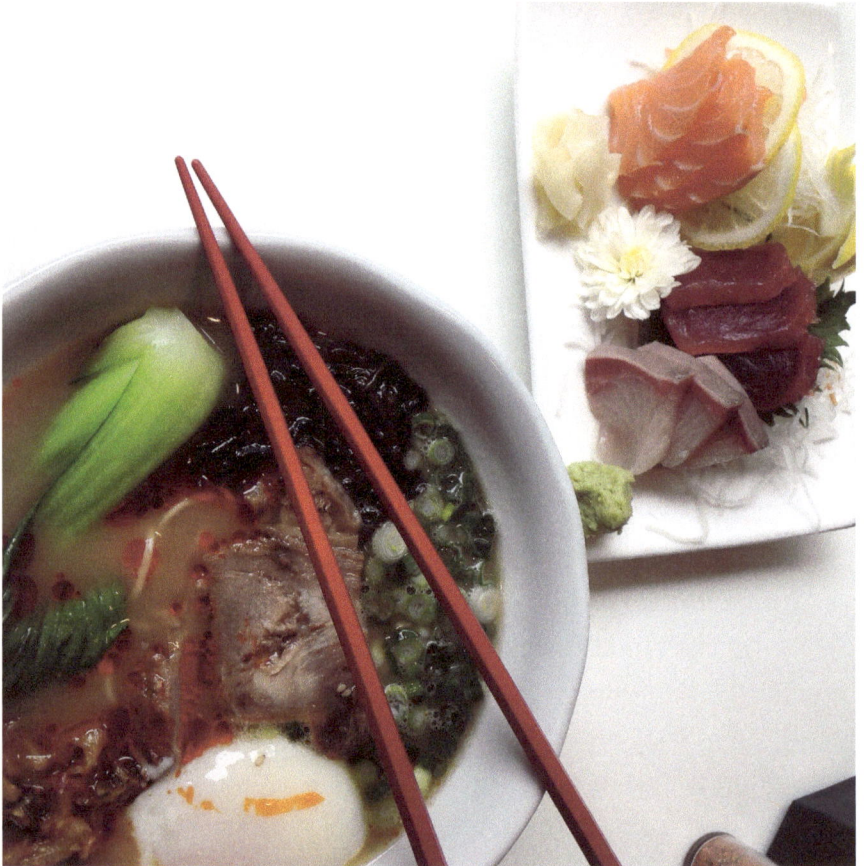

One much-neglected product is coconut oil. This got some bad press years ago as it is considered a saturated fat as it is solid at room temperature in the UK. However, it is abundant with medium chain triglycerides and specifically lauric acid. Whilst this last is a saturated fat it is now agreed that it generally improves blood cholesterol profiles by increasing the good HDL proportion. So substituting coconut oil for your usual vegetable oil for cooking is most definitely a good idea.

For some, the very mild coco-nutty flavour may not be to their liking but personally, I find it delicious.
Coconut oil is definitely one of the good fats and has been shown to improve cholesterol balance in the blood.

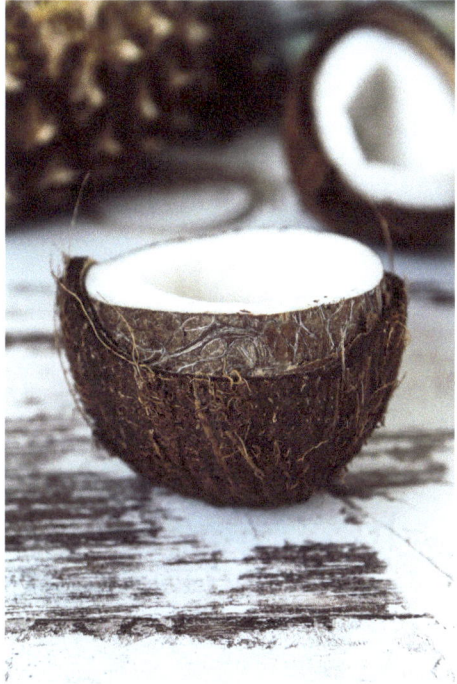

Diet drinks/aspartame

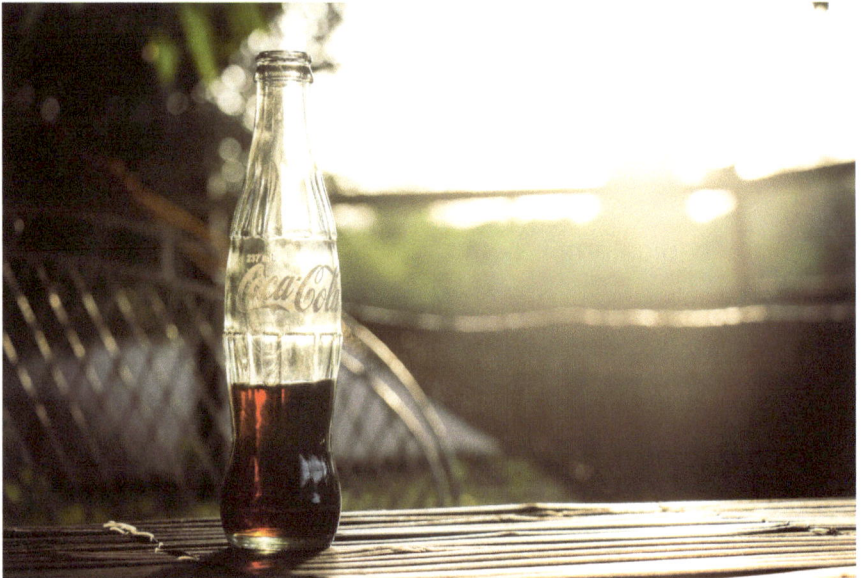

Whilst we are in the low fat section let me cover diet drinks and aspartame. First up this, by its nature, is very much an artificial chemical rather than a food. So black mark there then. And yes before I get a chorus from all the scientists out there, I know everything is a chemical in some form or other. A carrot freshly pulled from the ground is stuffed full of 'chemicals' no matter how organically it is grown, but I am attempting to separate naturally occurring chemicals in food that we have been dealing with for millennia from artificially created chemicals dreamed up by scientists in labs and made in factories. We should probably grow food rather than manufacture it….

So aspartame is an artificial chemical that fools our taste buds into thinking something is sweet. So why doesn't that sound like a good idea? Fewer calories and still a yummy taste.

Well when you consider that what we're trying to do is reduce insulin production, and insulin is primarily stimulated by dietary sugar and carbs, then this does seem like a good idea. We do however have to look a little more closely. Unfortunately, the process isn't that simple. If you give a person a sugary drink and then watch their blood levels of sugar and insulin then you do see a rise in both of these after the drink. However, you do see some insulin secretion prior to the rise in blood sugar. This is because the body has tasted the sweet drink and is thus anticipating the sugar rise. It, therefore, pre-empts this by kicking out some insulin early. This is an eminently sensible arrangement in the pre-industrial world to create a more stable sugar level. So the sweet taste alone stimulates some insulin production.

The now obvious drawback of this occurs when we drink our new "diet" soda. The body thinks it's about to get a sugar rise and so anticipates this with a small production of insulin. The sugar level does not rise (there were no calories after all) and instead falls due to the insulin. This insulin has done its storage job of putting whatever sugar is in your blood into the fat stores but unfortunately tends to make you more hungry due to the blood sugar drop.

Just think about that again for a second.

Does it help if I also mention that aspartame is added to some animal feeds to make them eat more and gain weight? Yes, the stuff in your diet coke is fed to animals to make them put on weight. If anyone doubts this effect can they just explain to me any other possible reason to put it in animal feed? I can't imagine the farmers want their cattle to loose weight.

It seems pretty unlikely to me that diet drinks can help weight loss very much. If anything it might just make you fatter. Does that sound like something you should be eating?

So I guess we're just going to have to get used to eating things a bit less sweet. Actually, as all food and diet is a habit you can get used to more and you can get used to less. Something to consider anyway. So if you are going to have any sweet stuff please get it from real food. So an actual strawberry as opposed to strawberry yoghurt, especially as the yoghurt has probably got added sugar as well.

Intermittent fasting

This is the main bit I have to thank Dr. Mosley for. This information about the latest research on fasting and calorie restriction truly revolutionised my life.
It has been known for a very long time that calorie restriction makes you live longer (It doesn't just make it seem longer…)
Back in the 20s and 30s lab experiments on mice showed that if you consistently fed mice on roughly 65% of their normal dietary intake they were not only healthier overall but lived significantly longer than their compatriots fed the normal diet.

Ever since that time, there have been a very determined group of humans who have persisted on a severely restricted human diet too with reasonable results (just a very boring life…).

More recent research has looked into other perhaps more acceptable ways to produce significant calorie restriction whilst maintaining a reasonable lifestyle. The latest research from Chicago is looking into alternate day fasting, so what does this involve?

Well, a true fast is when you go without any food and just drink water for a period of time. Many religions, over many

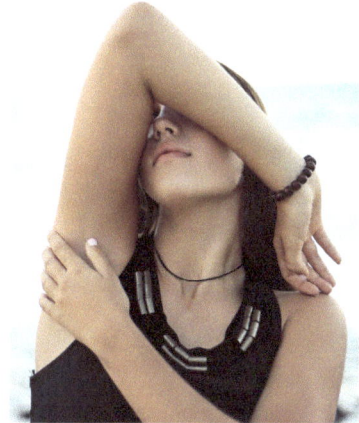

years, have recommended fasting to improve spiritual awareness. So there is a long history of doing this. In fact, if you go back to our ancestors crossing the African savanna you can see it as pretty normal.

These ancestors didn't live next to a Tesco express so you can pretty much guarantee they didn't have a regular three meals a day diet. In fact apparently even in roman times, the norm was for a very light breakfast of some kind of dried biscuit, working through lunch and then sit down for a 'proper' meal at night.

So to get back to our hunter-gatherer ancestors for a minute, they were a nomadic people with no fixed domicile. They would carry with them a small supply of dried fruit and nuts etc. They would gather whatever they could from the wild bushes etc and the men would hunt for whatever small game they could get hold of. Also big game too. They certainly would not have huge supplies of grains to make bread or pasta (no agriculture yet). So their overall calorie intake would be fairly low but when the men come home with a significant catch you have a very obvious problem.

Yes, you're right no fridge, so if you kill something substantial you need to eat all of it. The whole thing or else it'll go off pretty quick. So you can see that the whole feast/famine thing would be pretty damn normal.

Also whilst we're talking about them we need to point out that pickings in the winter would be even more scarce so it would be pretty important to put on some weight in the summer to get you through the lean times in the winter. So a fairly obvious corollary of this would explain why fruit can make you gain weight.

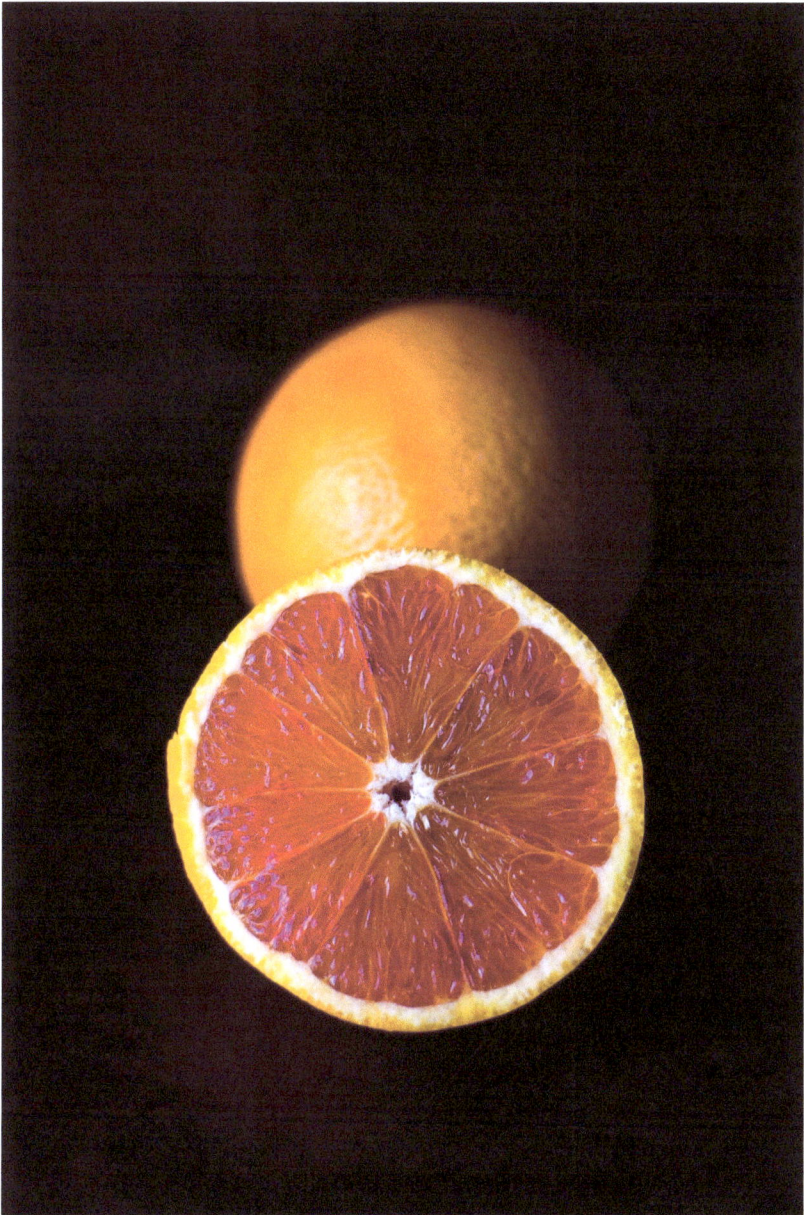

Conventionally fruit comes at the end of the summer. What happens after that is the winter, so eating a lot of fruit would signal to your body that winter was on its way you'd better put on some weight fast to get you through it. So whilst fruit does have a lot of vitamins and things in, we probably shouldn't eat too much. Back to the rainbow food thing again I guess.

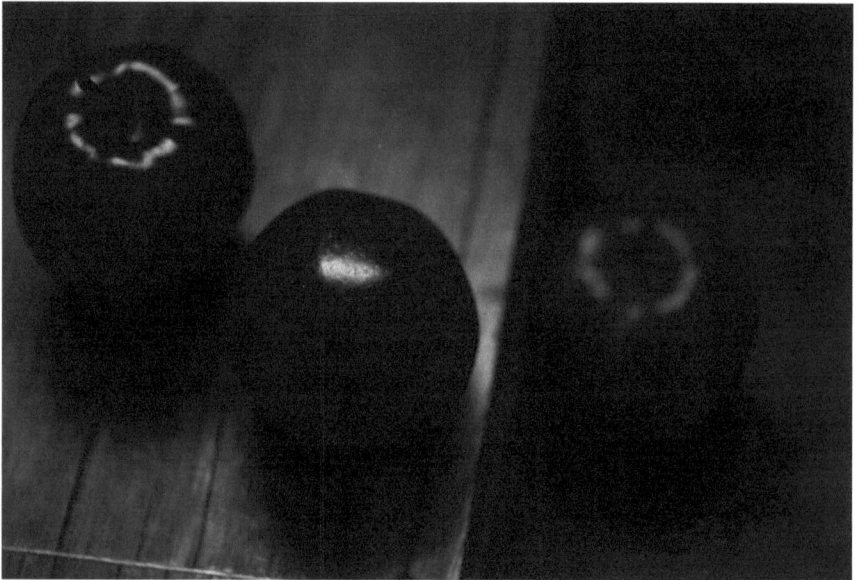

Anyway, I digress, over the years since the 30s the medical profession has suggested various forms of fasting as being beneficial to the body as well as the soul. I recently read a book by Dr. Edward Dewey from Philadelphia in the early 20th century. He was recommending complete water fasts for several days as a cure for pretty much everything. Now I always worry when someone suggests that anything can cure everything but he certainly had anecdotes from people who had gone several days to several weeks without any calories, just water.

Now I know the IRA hunger striker Bobby Sands lasted 66 days but he did die at that point so I am certainly not recommending anything like that but plenty of research has gone into fasting on just water for between 5 and 7 days.

This is still not the most pleasant thing to do with participants reporting headaches and naturally fairly severe hunger for the first few days. Interesting enough this hunger abates after the first few days and those who have fasted for longer have reported very little hunger.

Dr. Mosley however was recommending a gentler form of fasting in which a very small amount of calorie intake was allowed. He specifically recommends 25% and keeping that to only a single day.

This is where the methods digress somewhat and the Chicago study recommended alternate day reduction to 25% of normal calorific intake. Interestingly the research suggests that it doesn't matter much what you eat on the 'normal' days. More specifically they have looked into both high fat and low-fat versions of the normal days and seen no appreciable difference in effect. This is very interesting indeed.

So let's be more specific and do the maths on this one. If we take the usual intake for ladies as our example because the maths is simpler, we get 2000 calories per day as the recommended normal intake for most women. Yes, I know this recommendation takes no account of exercise etc but bear with me on this.

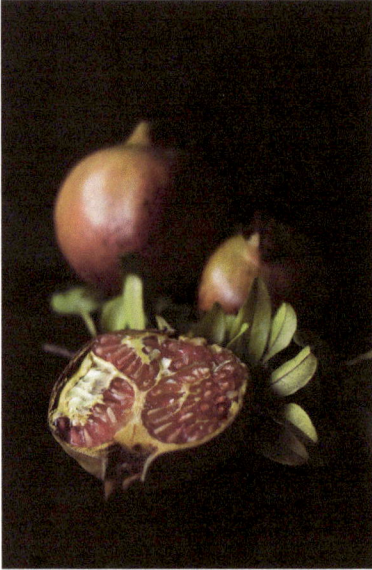

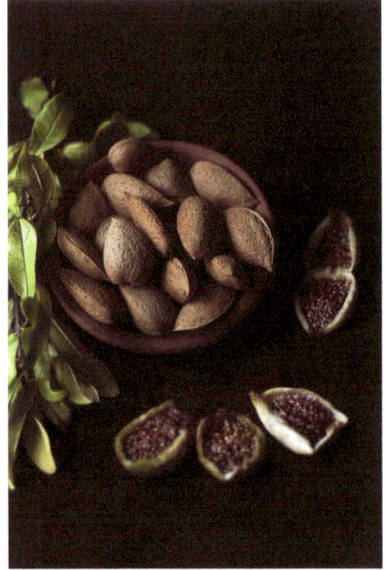

So 2000 calories per day equate to 14000 calories per week (2000 x7). If on only 3 days that week you eat just 25% of the usual intake i.e 500 calories then the overall calorific intake for that week would drop dramatically to 9500 (3x500 + 4x2000). Notice this is a 32% drop in total calories for the week leaving a residual of 68% (nearly that used in the previous mouse study).

They also went on to an even more interesting study when they compared two groups, one doing the alternate day fasting and the other doing the 68% calorific intake daily. So both groups consumed the same number of calories over the week but the first group was on the 'diet' every day whilst the others only had to do their more severe 'diet' only three days a week. The other four days they were told to eat what they wanted.

Interesting both groups lost weight and the differences were not significant. However, the alternate day group had physiological benefits over and above the weight loss that the other group didn't have.

This suggested that there was some extra benefit from going on a more severe restriction in a pulsatile manner.

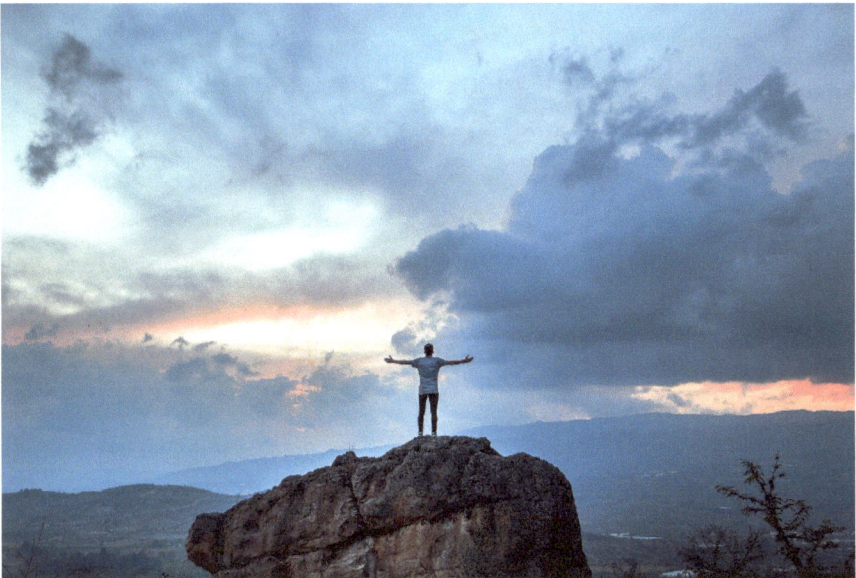

Also interestingly whilst some ladies reported on the trial that they preferred to take their 500 calories evenly spaced out through the day, the blood tests suggested that it was actually more beneficial to skip breakfast and lunch and have a small 500 calorie evening meal instead. There is, however, some more recent research that suggests there may be differences between men and women in their reaction to fasts and thus the recommendations may be different for each sex. However, the data for this is sketchy. I suppose you can just try it and see what works best for you.

Hold on a second I can hear some at the back, what about this bit about eating whatever you want on your 'normal' or non-fasting days?

Well, that's exactly the reason I like the alternate day version.

If you think about it for a second and you eat only 500 calories on Monday what's to stop you eating 3500 calories on Tuesday and blowing the whole deal?

Well, nothing, actually other than the fact that it is quite hard to do. No, it's not impossible but 3500 calories is a lot of food. A medium Dominoes pizza Pepperoni Passion with stuffed crust is 299 calories a slice so if you can manage to wolf down a whole 10 slices then you're getting there but as you can see that would be pretty hard to do. If you then start onto a curry with rice and Naan bread then you will probably have made it but I suspect you'd feel pretty full by then. So not impossible but not easy.

So what do I say to my patients which gets it in a nutshell?

On Monday skip breakfast and lunch (try to do this on a busy day, it's easier then) and have a five or six hundred calorie light evening meal.

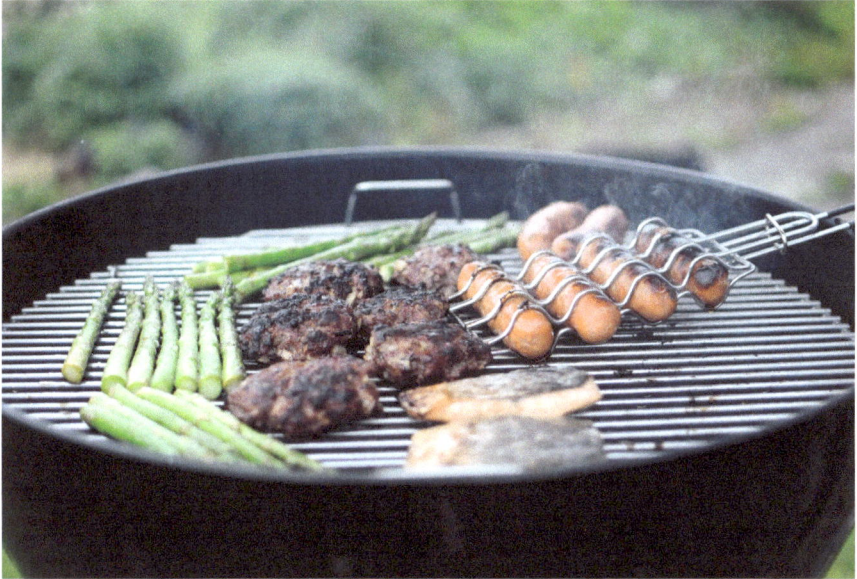

On Tuesday eat whatever you want to eat, but….. And yes it's a big BUT (to help you lose the big BUTT)

Eat what you want not what you think is good for you.
Stop eating as soon as you are no longer hungry.
Never get 'full'

Don't eat it because:-
- You paid for it.
- It's on the plate.
- Your grandma said you had to clean the plate.
- It's breakfast time (or lunch time etc.)
If you are hungry eat. If you are not, don't.

On your 'normal' days don't be hungry but don't ever get full.
Yes, that was worth repeating.

Why do we use our mouths like a bin and put the last bit on the plate in our mouths rather than in the bin?????
If you are no longer hungry, stop!

So to recap probably the best way to do alternate day fasting is to skip breakfast and lunch on your 'fast' day and simply have a light evening meal. (500 calories for women and 625 for men, yes I know its not fair, but there you go.) On your 'normal' days eat what you like.

5/2 version

Dr. Mosley preferred the 5/2 version for his own diet and there's nothing wrong with that. This boils down to only doing the 25% fast on two days a week. There is a slight downside as you do need to eat reasonably well on the other days or else it would be very easy to make the difference back up. If I remember rightly Michael also did prefer to evenly spread his calories throughout the day but it is worth remembering that most of the science suggests there is an added benefit to spending 16 to 24 hours with no food at all just water and remember if after your evening meal on a fast day you still feel hungry you can have a good breakfast tomorrow which doesn't seem too bad now does it?

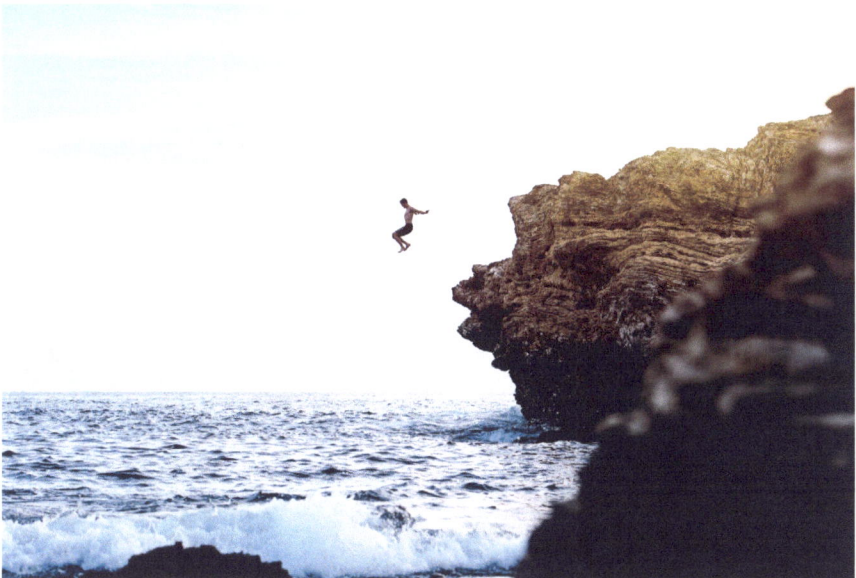

On the subject of hunger let me add another point. No one ever died of hunger. People have certainly died of starvation but as said earlier once you have not eaten anything for several days the hunger seems to disappear. So no matter how unpleasant you may think it is hunger is never going to do you any harm, so, so what. Just think how much good this new way of eating is doing for you.

One other thing which is worth saying is that all these versions of intermittent fasting form a spectrum of eating that you can place yourself on at any point and feel free to move up and down this spectrum as much as you like. As I said at the beginning this is no 'one size' fits all plan. Find what works for you. An obvious question might be what is the minimum amount of fasting you can do to gain the physiological benefits even if you no longer need to lose weight. Well the good news, again from the Chicago study, is it looks like it would be a good idea to fast roughly every 9 days. Making the process easier to remember once a week would be fine.

So if this wondrous diet plan that can improve your blood pressure, reduce your insulin resistance, improve you leptin resistance and make you live longer boils down to eventually once a week skipping breakfast and lunch that sounds pretty easy doesn't it?

Exercise

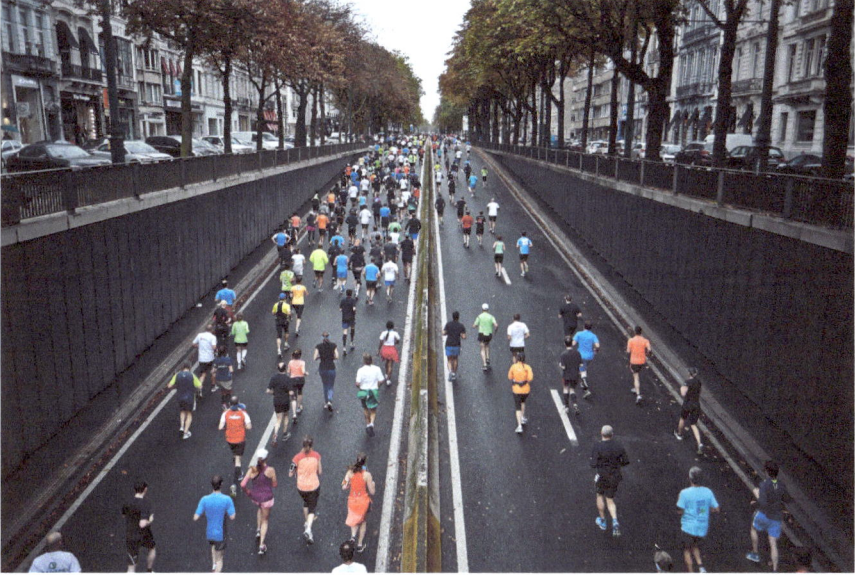

So lets deal with the other half of the equation. Calories in minus calories out equals gain or lose weight depending on the maths. Eat more than you do, gain weight. Do more than you eat, lose weight.

Yes, there are people out there now screaming that the calorie equation isn't the only relevant calculation. Quality and type of calories do matter, but you can't break the law of conservation of energy. This states that "Energy can be neither created nor be destroyed, but it transforms from one form to another, for instance, chemical energy can be converted to kinetic energy."

Thus the chemical energy in your food must either be transformed into kinetic energy by movement etc or converted into some other form of stored chemical energy i.e. fat. So in order to lose weight, more specifically to lose fat, you need to either eat less than you do or do more than you eat or preferably both.

The difference that quality and type of food makes is primarily in satiety and physiological responses which make you eat more or less.

So whilst fat loss is not completely dependent on exercise(and you can, of course, lose weight without doing any exercise), health, fitness and longevity do benefit from a reasonable level of exercise.

As this bit often gets confused I would like to make it clear. Diet is paramount. You cannot exercise away a poor diet. Teenagers can get away with it for a while for hormonal reasons, but adults over 30 become increasingly subject to their diet. Having said that from a strict longevity point of view there are very many hormonal and physiological reasons why 'reasonable' amounts of exercise are vital. Certainly, from an evolutionary standpoint, we are probably more sedentary now than we have ever been in the past, but the most important part of this discussion is the term 'reasonable'.

Very frequently when I ask my patients how much exercise they do they begin by making excuses about why it's not much at the minute but it either was plenty before or will be plenty after the procedure. The commonest reason people give for not doing 'enough' is a lack of time. This is I think because people seem to think that you need to spend at least an hour a day in the gym five days a week to be doing 'enough'!

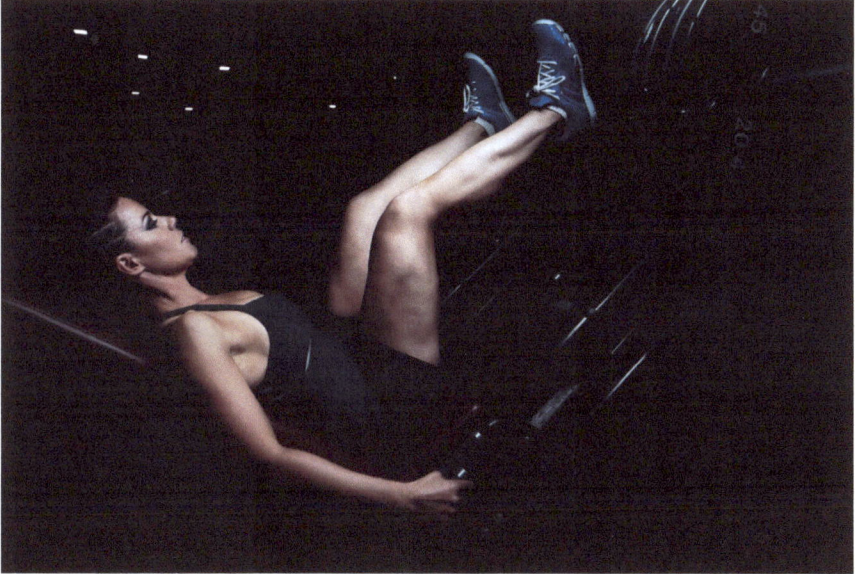

The really good news here is you really don't need to do anything like that much. Some of the latest studies show improvements in cardiovascular fitness and an increase in lung efficiency with as little as 10 to 20 minutes of high-intensity interval training twice a week. One study even suggested that it was enough to go flat out for 30 seconds pause briefly and repeat twice just once a week. The important factor here is intensity. It is mostly about the amount of effort put in. What exactly is 'flat out'?

Any exercise you can sustain for 50 plus minutes cannot be 'flat out'. We are talking sprints here not marathons.

In fact, this leads me to my next illustration. In your mind's eye picture two Olympic athletes, a marathon runner and a sprinter. Undeniably both are very fit. Which one would you rather look like?

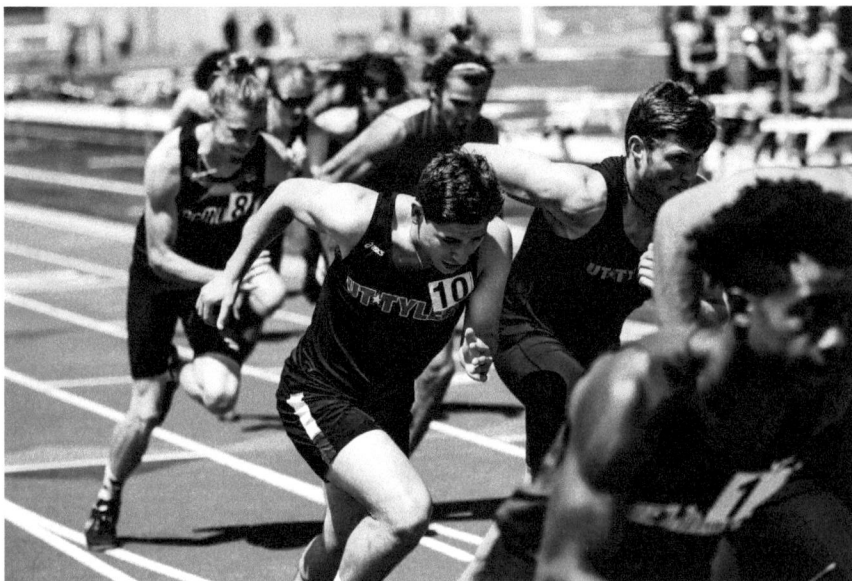

On average most sprinters are muscular toned individuals with an excellent looking physique whilst most marathon runners are thin and lanky and not necessarily very 'healthy' looking. With this in mind can you please explain to me whilst those people keen on starting an exercise regime tend to begin with hour-long gentle to moderate 'aerobics' sessions.

I know this is a major generalisation here but there are two kinds of people in the UK with relation to exercise. Those that don't do any (the majority) and those that probably do too much.

So remember we are talking sprints here so you absolutely don't need to spend at least an hour doing a spin class or aerobics superclass or anything similar. I am not saying these are necessarily bad for you. (Some most certainly are and one recent one called 'Insanity training' really lives up to its name) But they most certainly aren' t the most efficient way to spend you precious few available exercise 'moments'.

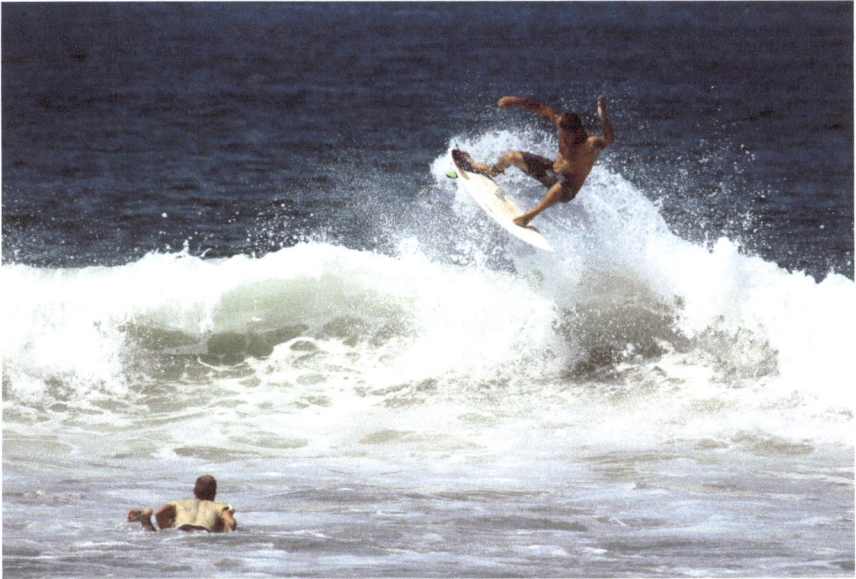

Several recent studies have shown high levels of traumatic joint damage to long distance runners and the well-documented cases of unfortunate charity marathon runners who have collapsed and died whilst running must give one pause for thought. You have to also remember that the reason most exercise classes are roughly an hour is purely down to easy scheduling. There is no scientific evidence to suggest that unless you exercise for an hour you're not doing enough.

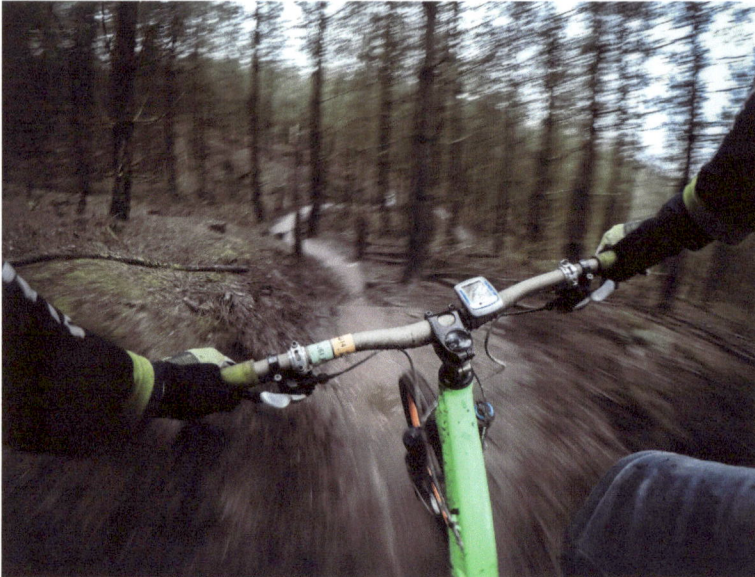

So how much exercise do we really need and what is the most efficient way to get it?

Several recent studies now indicate that the most important aspect of any exercise regime is intensity rather than duration. One particular study suggests that as little as three 30 second episodes of 'flat out' exercise done twice per week are enough to improve lung function and cardiovascular health.

I usually suggest a high-intensity interval program which involves 3 minutes of warm up followed by 30 seconds of flat out, followed by 90 seconds of coasting, followed by 30 seconds of flat out….etc. Repeat between 5 and 8 times. This approximates to 13 to 20 minutes of cardiovascular exercise repeated twice weekly.

The most important bit, however, is the definition of 'flat out'. A simple description is just as fast as you can, but to be more precise, if you can do whatever you are doing for even 2 or 3 minutes then you aren't going fast enough. I normally say 30 seconds sprints but if you are really going 'flat out' you should probably be struggling at 20 seconds or so and get to say 27 absolutely gasping to stop. That would be my definition of flat out. The interesting aspect of this is this is not a particular speed or distance it is a measure of effort. Thus when you start out it may not be very fast or over a particularly long distance but as you get fitter and still put the same intensity of effort in then you will naturally be going faster and covering more distance in the same time.

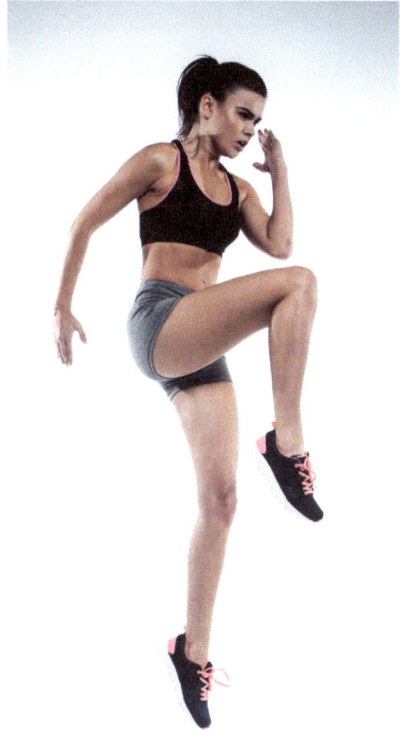

This regime will get you the maximum cardiovascular benefit in the minimum of time and thus pretty much anyone can fit this into their schedule no matter how busy they may be. So that deals with the cardiovascular bit but you do need to do some muscle work too.

Let's get this out of the way from the start. We all benefit from some weight training. Weight training tones muscles and can help to build muscles. Bigger muscles burn more calories just sitting still, so they help burn off the fat if you need to lose weight. Also being stronger just makes most of life easier anyway. But I know many ladies will shy away from weight training because they don't want to look like Arnold Schwarzenegger.

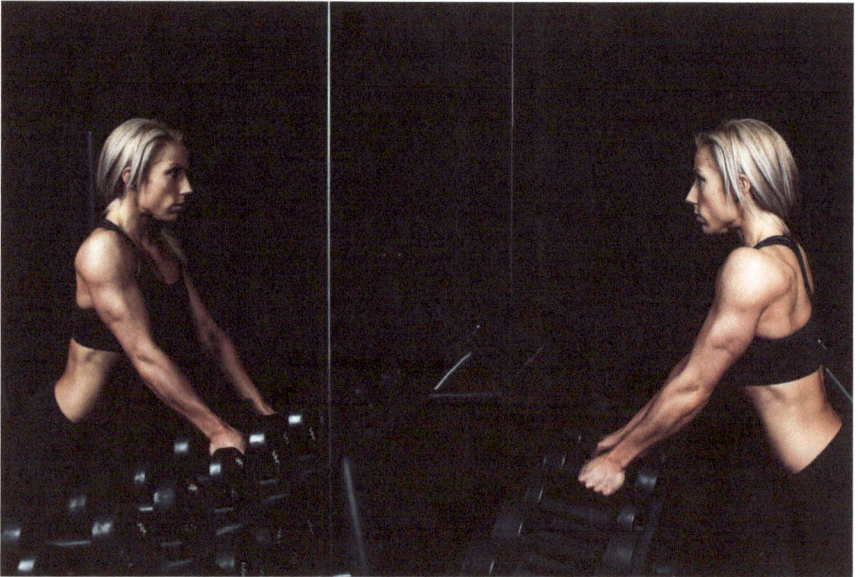

Ladies, you won't ever look like Arnold. Even dedicated body-building ladies don't get close despite the most stringent of diets and massively extended exercise plans (and maybe some steroids too). Even Arnold probably used a whole load of supplements and stimulants to get like he did. Having said that ladies arms look more shapely with a little bit of extra muscle. And the extra strength might well help you open that stubborn jar lid too.

But here is another conundrum. Most ladies who do weights do high repetition low weight exercises. Well sorry ladies, but that is just aerobics with weights.

What I am talking about here is low repetition high weight exercise. Once again it comes down to intensity. We are mostly looking for exercise until 'failure'. In other words, repeat the movement until you feel you really can't do anymore. So when conventionally people recommend 3 sets of 8 reps, then the first set should be reasonable, the second should be a little hard and the last 2 or 3 reps of the third set would be almost impossible. In fact, I would go so far as to say if you can't complete the third set due to absolute muscle exhaustion then that probably means you picked the right weight.

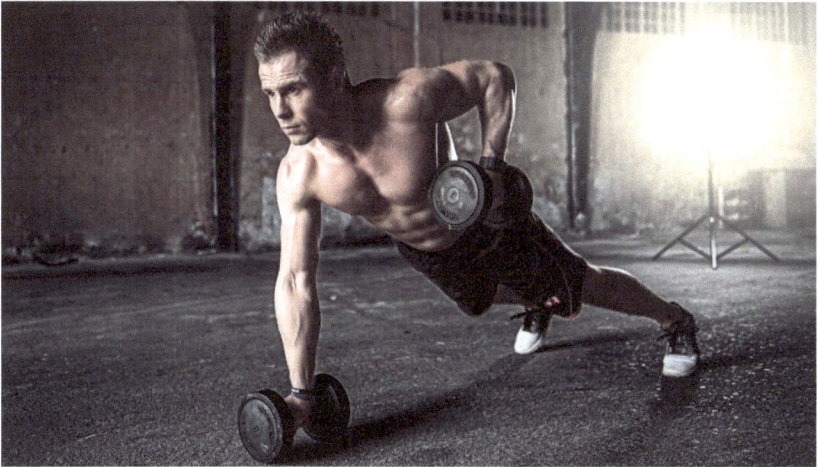

If you can do 3 sets of 8 easily then you are not using nearly enough weight.

To take this to its extreme you can perform a static contraction exercise with a single rep. One way to do this is to pick the most weight you can just about hold for 7 seconds. Now if you can't pick it up at all then that's too much, but if you can hold it for 20 seconds then it is not enough.

Another important principle in this is every time you exercise you must beat your previous weight. So if last time you lifted 10kg this time it must be 12kg.

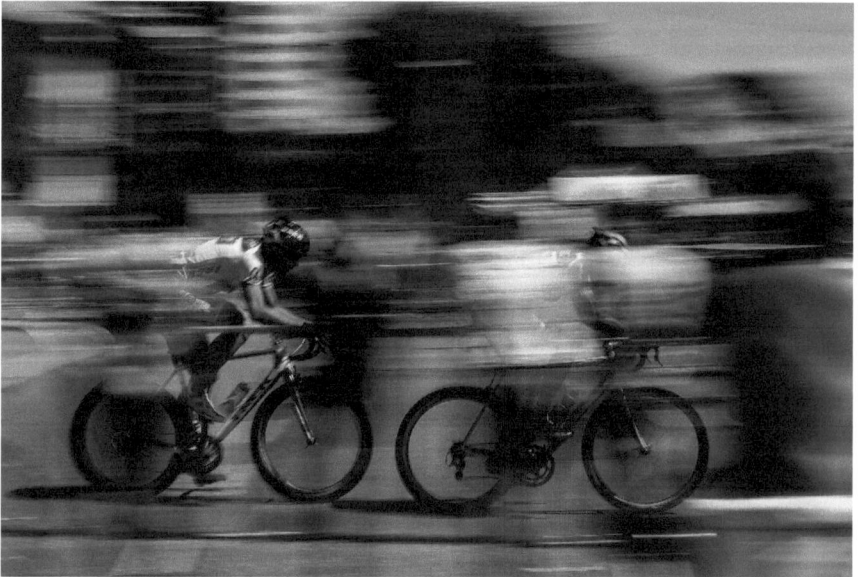

We then get into discussing how often you need to do the weight training sessions. Again increasing new studies have turned the standard recommendations on their heads.
Most body building gym freaks insist on three times a week, say Monday, Wednesday, Friday. This is fine at the beginning but often after a while they find they struggle to continue to make further strength improvements. Remember you have to beat your target from the last session.

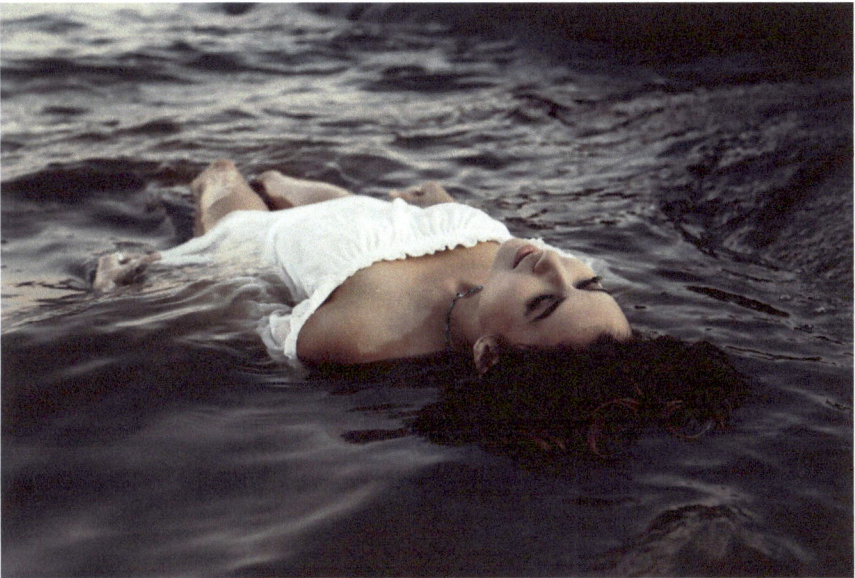

So lets say you do Monday, Wednesday, Friday for several weeks and each time you are getting better, eventually one of the sessions will see a plateau and you can't beat the previous one. Conventional wisdom will say you're not trying hard enough or your diet must be wrong or something else is going on. However, recent studies have suggested that you are just not getting enough rest between sessions.

Yes, I said that right you need to get more rest. You need to give your body time to recover from the intensity of the previous session. So instead of Monday, Wednesday, Friday, you might need to skip Wednesday and just do Monday, Friday.
Surprisingly you will discover that by having a missed day you will actually be stronger on Friday and thus able to beat Monday's scores again.

After a few more weeks of this you may well reach another plateau and thus need to skip another exercise day and just do once a week. In this way, in some studies, guys working at very high levels got down to doing their weight training episodes once every 6 weeks but on each and every occasion they were able to improve on their previous results. Let me repeat that this was doing a single all out rep for each movement so the whole weight training session could be as little as 5 to 10 minutes every six weeks. This was at a very intense level and working hard in this way at one time I had my leg press figures up to 814 lb which is roughly four times my body weight.

So this really does work and again can provide maximum physiological benefit in the smallest amount of our precious time.

As a general guide, I suggest people do a minimum of one maximally intense weight training session a week for build up and then also maintenance.

So in summary then, do two high intensity interval training sessions a week of roughly 15 to 20 minutes. Three minutes warm up followed by 30 seconds 'flat out', followed by 90 seconds 'cool down' followed by another 30 seconds 'flat out' etc repeating between 5 and 8 times.

Once a week, do a super efficient weight training session to build and tone muscle. If you want to look better then increase the scores each session. If you are happy with how you look then maintain the figures to maintain the results.

One additional way of improving the efficiency of the weight training is to do 'super slow' sets. So if you are doing biceps curls and wish to do 3 sets of 8 then take at least 10 seconds over every movement. Five down and five up for example. This super slow movement engages all the different muscle fibres and again maximises benefits. Again intensity is King and so you need to push yourself to repeat the movements until you feel totally unable to do anymore. If this is 30 or 40 reps then you need more weight.

Whilst we are on the subject of exercise we need to make a mention of 'non-exercise related movement'. Recent studies have suggested that simply spending less time sitting down or lying down can have beneficial effects even if no formal exercise regime is in place. So making sure to get up roughly every 45 minutes at work and spend a bit of time walking around and stretching your legs is a good idea. Try

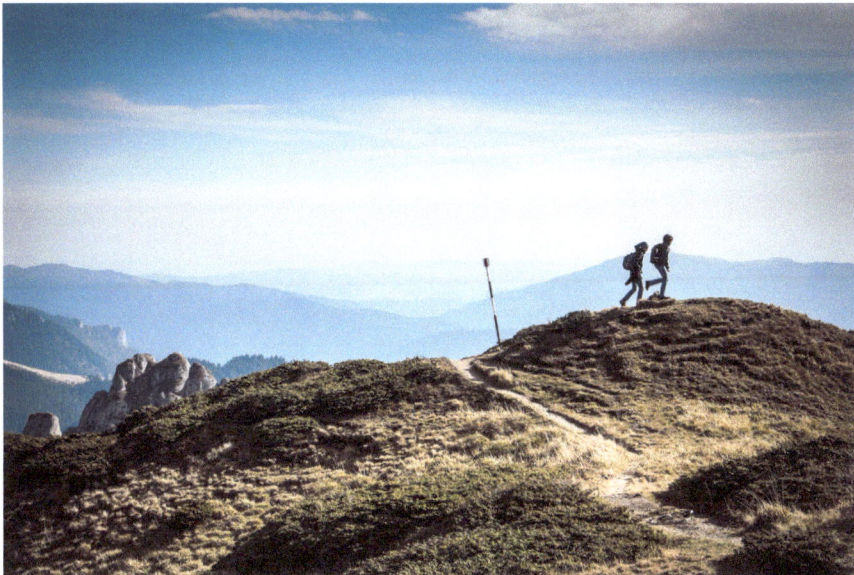

incorporating a few simple squats and touching your toes will also help.

Taking the stairs rather than the lift or escalators is also important and the general aim of trying to get at least 10,000 steps per day is a good place to start. I do highly recommend a pedometer of some sort not only to assess what you are doing but also because having one tends to change what you do and make you more aware of opportunities to 'get your steps in'. Another suggestion is significant manual labour whether it is chopping logs for the fire or digging in the garden these all add to your exercise regime without feeling like exercise at all.

Drink more water

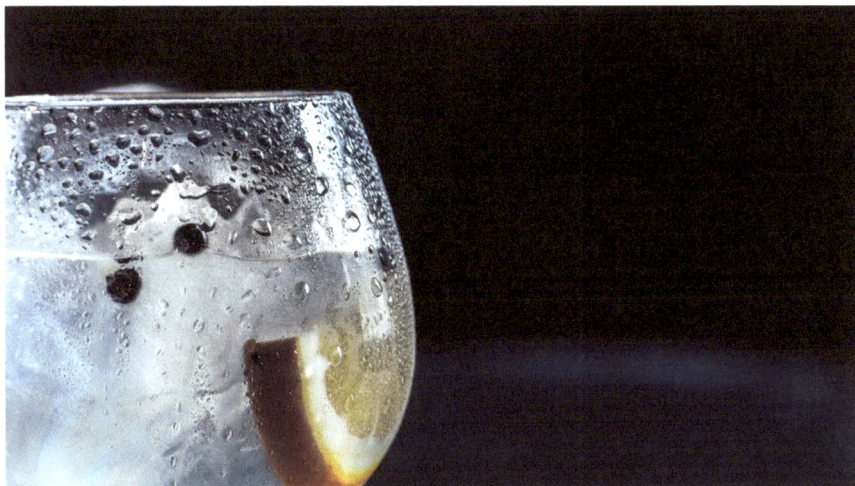

Now, I worried a great deal when I wrote out this chapter heading because there is a lot of controversy about this and some people do take it to extremes. So I am going to take it slowly and spell out my own personal view of the myths and legends about water. Please feel free to extensively research this yourself and come to your own opinions. Suffice it to say that in my own research I have changed my opinions over the years quite a few times.

Anyway, water. Probably the most important thing for life after oxygen.

You can only survive several minutes without oxygen, several days without water and several weeks without food. Of course, similarly you can have too much oxygen, and hyperbaric chambers where you can therapeutically use higher concentrations of oxygen have to be carefully monitored to prevent the toxic oxygen effects. You most certainly can have too much water, either by drowning or more appropriately you can develop a condition known as Diabetes Insipidus which is related to toxic levels of water consumption. This often leading to various chemical imbalances in the blood such as hyponatraemia which is a condition of low sodium levels.

Finally, you can, of course, have too much food which is a condition we all know far too well as that is why we are reading this book. Well, you are reading it and I am writing it but let's not get too pedantic.

There have been various views about what is the right amount of water to drink and some would advocate at least two litres a day. Not all of this needs to be drunk as there is a lot of water in our food. Some others have advocated even higher levels of water consumption and this is where we get into difficult areas. You need to take into account the environment where you live, (increase water consumption in a hot environment) the amount of exercise you do, and this all needs to be carefully balanced with the amount of sodium in your diet.

Keep in mind that in those unfortunates who have collapsed and died during charity marathon runs the major cause of death has been from cardiac arrhythmias related to the hyponatraemia brought on probably by drinking too much water during the event.

The adult male human body contains between 55-75% water but this varies considerably with sex, age, weight and physical fitness. Fat contains 10% water and muscle more like 75%. The obese therefore tend to have a lower water percentage and this is the basis of those electronic scales which estimate your body fat percentage depending on electrical impedance.

Unfortunately, the daily water recommendations also vary considerably and this must make it hard to know what to do. The most famous adage is drink 8 eight ounce cups of water a day and this equates to about 1.9 litres. Other recommendations vary between two and three litres a day. I have even seen some extreme recommendations much higher than this.

Water is essential for life. It provides the medium for chemical reactions in your cells, it provides the transport for fuel and oxygen around your body. You naturally secrete water back into the environment all the time via your sweat, your urine and even the moisture vapour in your breath so this all needs to be regularly replaced. Some have argued that if you wait until you are thirsty then you are already mildly dehydrated. On this point, there is not necessarily agreement by the majority.

There is, however, one physical sign you can check at frequent intervals which will give you quite a good guide to how well you are doing.

Urine.

If you regularly check the colour and relative volume (no I don't need you to pee in a measuring cup) of your output whenever you go you get a good general guide to your state of hydration.

You should aim to pass reasonable volumes of pretty clear urine. A little yellow is ok but try to get it as clear as possible most of the time. This would indicate that your body has plenty of fluid input.

Also remember that we are not only considering drinks as a lot of foods contain a lot of water. Soups, obviously, but also most fruit and vegetables contain considerable water volumes. Watermelon, for example, is almost 90% water. So the urine colour is actually a good indicator of hydration and a good guide to how much fluid you need.

Keep in mind that the amount you need to drink will depend also on your activity levels and your local weather so when it is hot or when you are exercising you'll need more. You also need to consider salt input if you are sweating a lot as you will be losing electrolytes from your body in the sweat.

Having raised the issue of salt and other electrolytes we need to discuss what to drink too.

The most thirst-quenching thing is plain water, but often this is thought of as boring. Unfortunately, pretty much everything you add to the water to make it less boring doesn't add to the nutritional value and some things are positively a bad idea.

So to go back to the sweeteners discussion briefly can I please, gently, ask you to refrain from all sodas and 'fizzy' drinks. Whether 'diet' or otherwise, these are all pretty bad for you for all the reasons we have previously discussed.

Things which can be added to water which are either neutral or possibly beneficial include, lemon juice (a squeeze of a quarter or eighth in a glass), black coffee (caffeinated arguably better than decaf, but needs further discussion), green tea, black tea (preferably without milk and definitely without sugar) and various 'herbal teas' if you like that sort of thing.

Unfortunately adding milk and sugar to any of them is a bad idea. Most fruit juices are a bad idea as they have too much sugar in them, even those with 'no added sugar'. Even naturally occurring fruit sugars can be too much.

Supplements

I don't really want to say a lot about supplements for two main reasons.

1.	The media are full of recommendations and the health food stores are simply overflowing with stuff.
2.	I would, however, prefer you to get most of your nutrition from good old fashioned wholesome food.

Having said that there is some suggestion that the quality of food now available from the supermarket is not as nutritious as it once was due to agricultural practices and the supermarket's desire for appearance and shelf life priorities.

There are some vitamins which have good evidence behind them to suggest a supplement may not be a bad idea. There is quite a good support for Vitamin B12, B6, and Folic acid supplementation as being helpful to maintain neurological function. Vitamin D is probably best obtained from the sun but those in the more northerly climes (including the UK) don't really get enough sun in the winter for adequate Vit D production so a supplement may be advised in the winter months.

Omega 3 supplementation is probably also worth recommending if you have an average western diet which tends to have a skewed Omega 3/Omega 6 balance. Arguably the cleanest form of omega 3 oils is from Krill which are harvested from antarctic seas and show very little evidence of industrial pollution.

There are lots of other herbs and vitamins which are specific for particular problems but I think as a general rule the ones above would be recommended and link this with the idea of 'rainbow' food and a prominence of natural 'living' food i.e. from the fridge rather than the cupboard.

Stay out of the sun

So I have probably just got myself into trouble by talking about Vitamin D and then saying stay out of the sun, so this will require more explanation.

Those living in more northern latitudes in the northern hemisphere (and naturally those living more southerly in the southern hemisphere) probably don't get enough sun exposure in the winter months to generate enough Vit D from this alone. So I recommend supplements in the winter months. But apart from that, elsewhere and everywhere in the summer it doesn't take very much sun exposure to generated enough vitamin D.

The recommendations vary a bit but I tend to believe that on a reasonably sunny day you can generate enough vitamin D on forearms exposed to direct sunlight for about an hour. The skin might go just a touch pink. You certainly don't need to expose your whole body and lie baking in the sun for several hours going bright red and risking sunburn.

So why do I say 'stay out of the sun'?

Facial ageing is indelibly linked to sun exposure. That is not to say that it is the only cause but it is a very significant one. This is a well-known picture of a truck driver from the states. You can see a massive difference in the wrinkles and other signs of ageing on the left side of his face. This was the side nearest the truck window and thus received the most UV exposure. So facial ageing is certainly significantly due to photo-damage or damage due to long exposure to ultraviolet light. So whilst vitamin D is undoubtedly very good for you, you are better off keeping your head out of the sun. As much as possible, whenever possible.

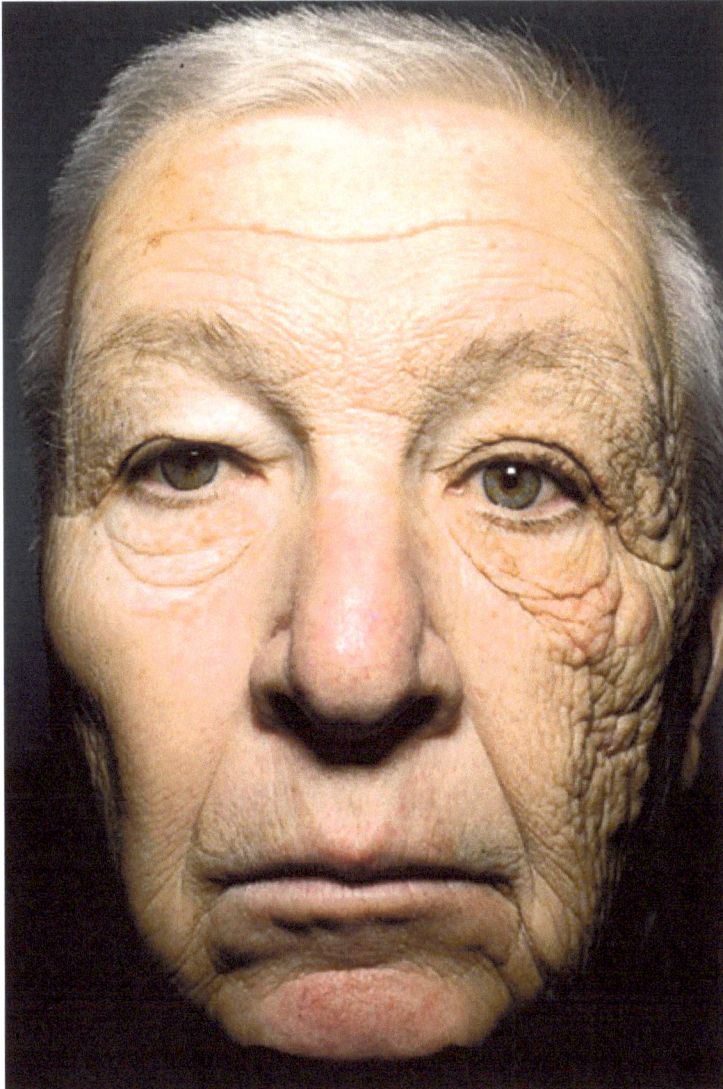

Get plenty of sleep

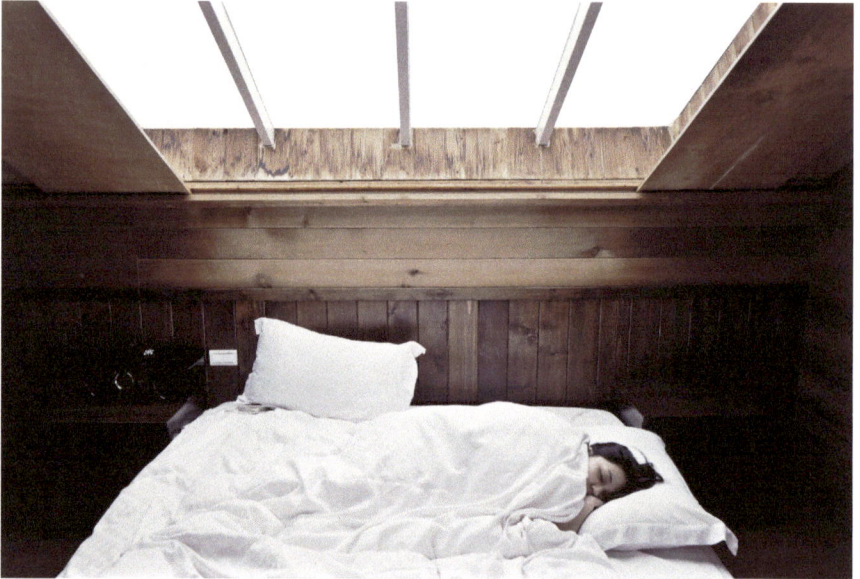

This does seem pretty obvious but there is some degree of debate about what constitutes plenty of sleep. During a single night, we all go through several cycles of deep and shallow sleep. Some of us are more aware of the shallow periods and some may believe that have been awake during some of these times. We tend to dream during these periods of shallow sleep, also known as REM sleep or Rapid Eye Movement sleep.

There is a lot of debate about the function of dreams and some think of them as pure entertainment for the brain during the rest period whilst others think of them as the way for the brain/mind to come to terms with psychological stresses treat have come up during the previous day. In an average 7 to 8-hour sleep session, there are only usually 3 to 4 periods of REM of roughly 30 to 45 minutes. These periods do appear however to be very important. In fact, if you shorten people's opportunity to sleep they tend to go into the REM state more quickly to in effect 'make sure they get it'. In fact in a significantly unpleasant test endured by some medical students they allowed them full access to sleep but woke them whenever they entered REM. Thus stopping them from effectively dreaming and several pointers of significant psychological stress appeared very quickly including some frank psychotic episodes. So whatever dreams are doing we absolutely need them.

There is more debate about exactly how long we need to sleep with most people recommending 7 to 8 hours but many examples of particularly famous people coping with very much less. Winston Churchill was said to only sleep one or two hours a night but coped by taking frequent cat naps during the day. Some reported these to be moments of meditation or self-hypnosis. Margaret Thatcher has been reported to cope admirably well on just 4 hours a night.

So we can undoubtedly manage with a lot less than 8 hours (which is lucky as most junior doctors used to have to) but what is optimum?

I believe there is significant individual variation in this and I am pretty convinced that being stressed about your apparent lack of sleep might, in fact, be more stressful than the actual lack of sleep. There is even some recent research into our dedication to eight straight hours being a fairly new phenomenon. Before the easy access to electric light we tended to go to sleep when it got dark and awake when the sun returned and down near the equator that is fairly regular but in the northern climes of Europe that can vary enormously at different times of the year with short nights in summer and long nights in winter. Apparently during the winter it may have been common to have two periods of sleep, the first soon after dark followed by a wakeful period in the middle of the night and then a further short sleep before daybreak. Certainly, shift work patterns can be significantly stressful and may be less than 'good for you'.

I personally feel that whilst there is some evidence to suggest that aiming for reasonable amounts of restful time on a regular 24 hour basis is certainly more healthful than a chaotic regime it is probably also true that most of us can cope perfectly well with the occasional disruption (from babies etc) we should probably try to worry less about how much sleep we actually get as can be seen from the next chapter stress in and of itself is a major contributor to the aging process and counter to good health.

Reduce stress

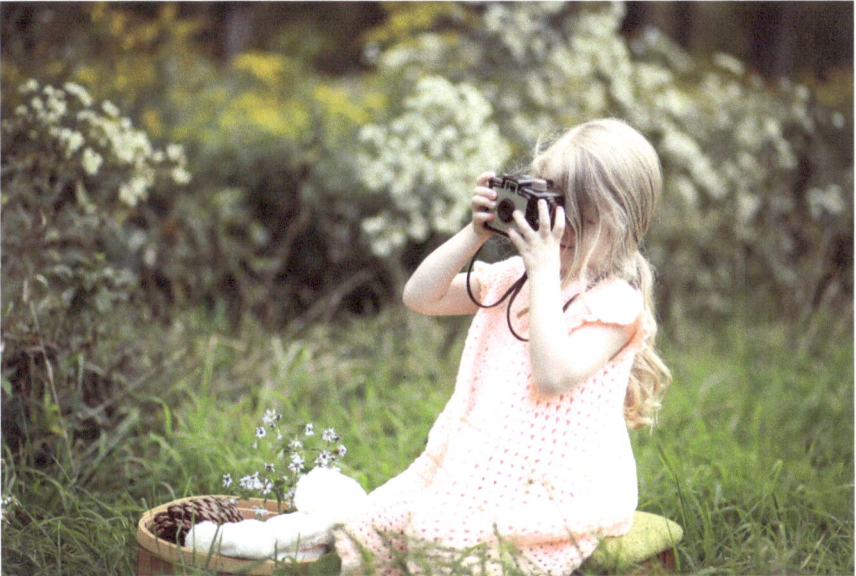

Let's talk about stress. Adrenaline and Cortisol are the main stress hormones and these are involved in the fight or flight principle. Adrenaline puts up your blood pressure and raises your heart rate. Cortisol is a steroid hormone which regulates a wide range of processes throughout the body including metabolism and the immune response. It also has a very important role in helping the body respond to stress. It promotes gluconeogenesis and increases the blood pressure amongst many other effects.

Whilst this may have been a great idea in the past if you were confronted by a lion or a marauding Viking, thus helping you stay alive on a short term basis. The fact is we are no longer frequently attacked by lions or Vikings and the more persistent or chronic stresses which we all have to deal with can be damaging to our metabolism and ultimately our health.

Now, funnily enough, I don't actually like the word stress, I prefer distress. That's because we all have different levels of stress which we seek out in our daily lives. We have all chosen or at least gravitated towards jobs, lifestyles and activities which produce different levels of stress. In fact, a certain amount of stress is necessary and healthy.

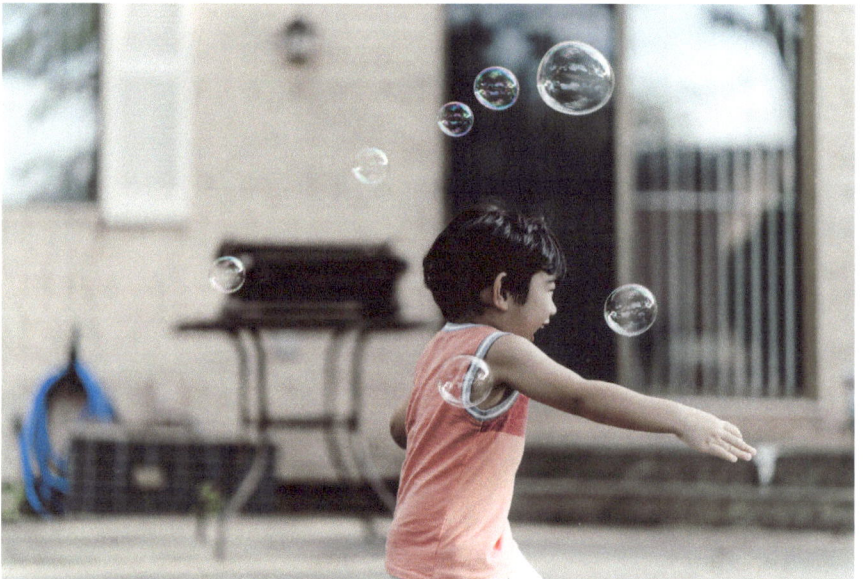

It is only when we stress our muscles in the gym or else-where that we stimulate muscle growth and gain strength. There is a thing called Hormesis. This is a biological phe-nomenon whereby a beneficial effect (improved health, stress tolerance, growth or longevity) results from exposure to low doses of an agent that is otherwise toxic or lethal when given at higher doses. This can refer to toxins (biological stressors) or actions (physiological stressors such as exercise).

So stress is not necessarily all negative. The important thing is how we respond or react to these stresses.
Some people seek out significant stress for entertainment such as scary movies or skydiving, so the term distress can be used for stress that is experienced by the individual in excess of that which is desired. Sorry if that sounds pedantic but it does help to clarify our definition and help guide us to what we can do about this distress.

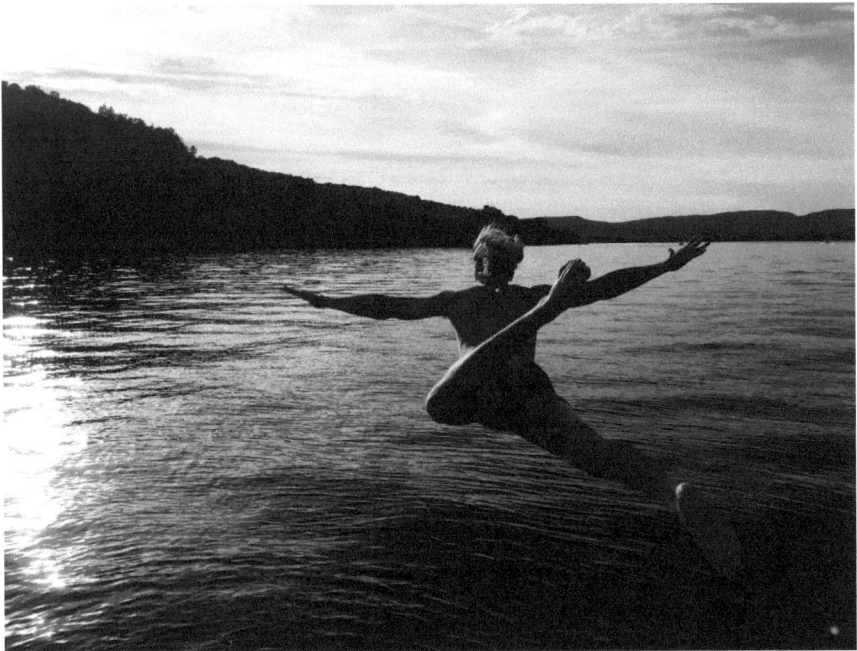

Firstly, of course, it depends what the causes of our stress are. So if you are in an unsatisfactory and depressing job or relationship then maybe you need to look seriously at what you can do to change the situation. Other problems might have less drastic solutions.

One thing I frequently shared with my GP patients was the Serenity Prayer of Reinhold Niebuhr which says:-

God, grant me the serenity to accept the things I cannot change, courage to change the things I can and wisdom to know the difference.

I have always declared this to be perfect stress management. In every stressful situation, there are things which cannot be changed. Often the hardest thing is to accept that and move on. Knowing what you can fix is crucial and then getting up and doing it completes the picture.

If you can divide your stresses into things you can cope with and things you want to change that can go a long way to making the world seem a better place.

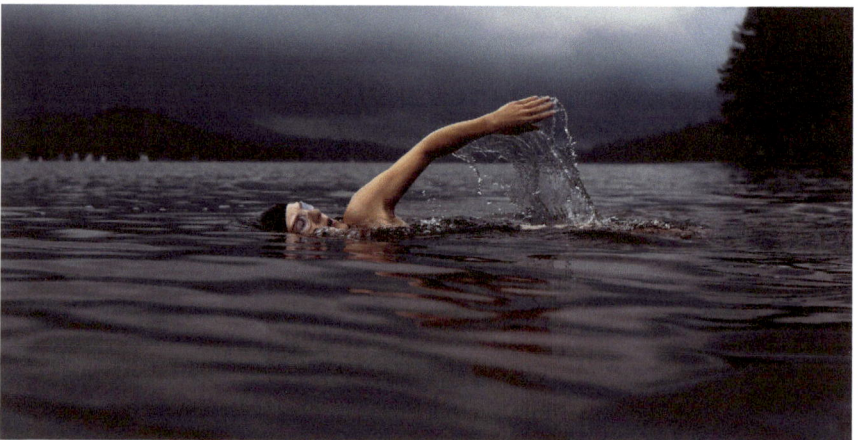

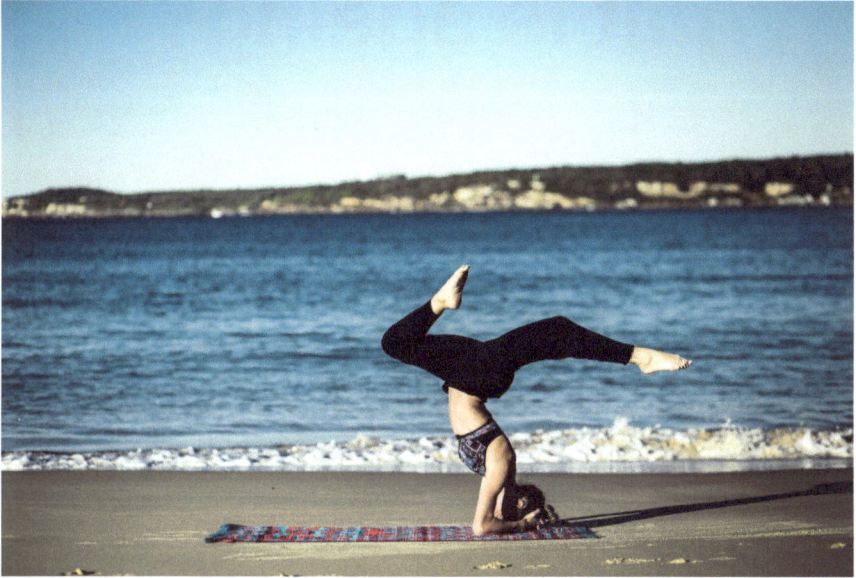

Other more practical things you need to consider are things like Yoga or Meditation which can certainly help with those aspects of the distress in your life that cannot be fixed.

Exercise too can be a great stress reducer. So fitting a regular exercise regime into your daily plan is always a good idea.

Undoubtedly stresses of all sorts can affect both the enjoyment and the duration of your time here on earth and so taking practical and simple steps to cope can make a big difference.

What is ageing?

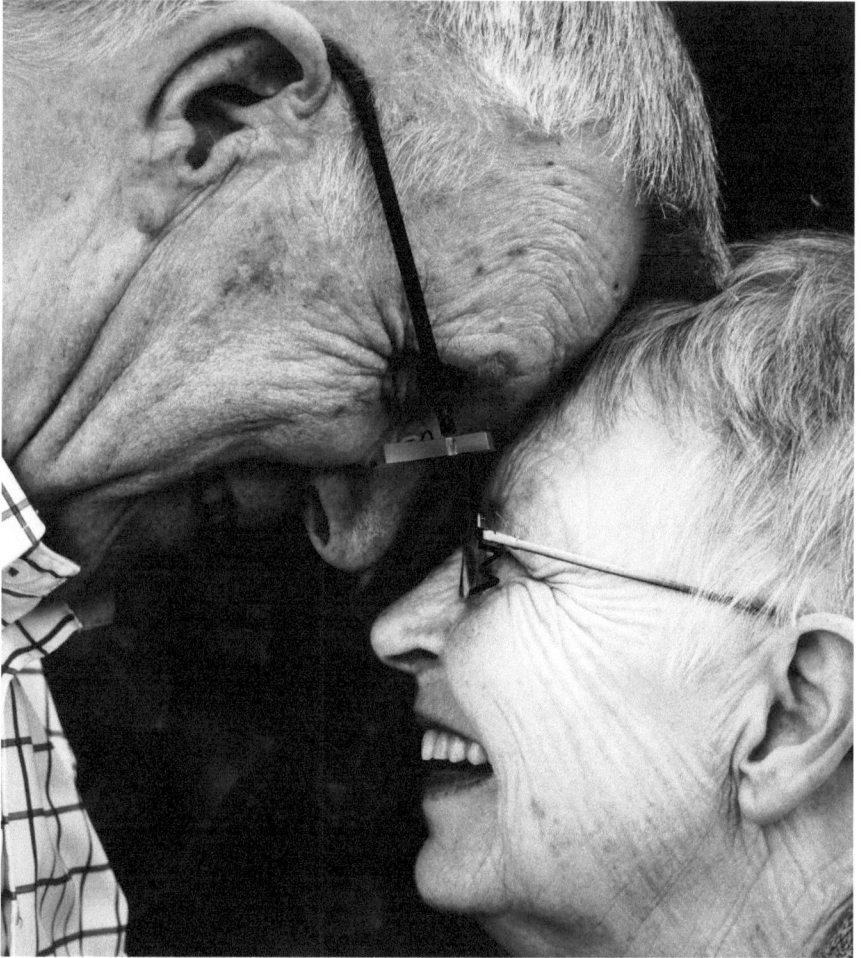

This may seem at first like a silly question but there are parts of the ageing process that appear to be inevitable and parts that appear to be more to do with lifestyle choices.

So if you look at a baby, a teenager, a parent and a grand-parent you can see obvious differences in physical characteristics. However, if you look at a group of grandparents you can see significant differences amongst them as well. Some seem to be 'better preserved' than others. As a cosmetic doctor myself I am very much aware of the treatments which can alter the outward appearance but here I am more concerned with both the physiological and the psychological differences that may be evident.

There does appear to be some sort of internal clock working and some sort of limit in possible longevity. Recent research has suggested that the longest we might be able to achieve is something like 120 years. It is mildly interesting to note that references to this sort of age limit actually occur in the bible so maybe they knew a bit more than they let on.....
This limit is physiological and something to do with the number of regenerative cycles that various organs and tissues in the body can reasonably undergo.

Just staying alive requires a turnover of cells as older less functional cells are replaced by new ones. This varies significantly depending on the type of tissue studied.

Red blood cells live for about four months, while white blood cells live on average more than a year. Skin cells live about two or three weeks. Colon cells have it rough: They die off after about four days. Sperm cells have a life span of only about three days, while brain cells typically last an entire lifetime (neurons in the cerebral cortex, for example, are not replaced when they die). So the body you live in today is not the body you had say 10 years ago but some of it probably is.

When I was in medical school we were definitely taught that you had as many neurons in the brain at roughly 13 as you were ever going to have. Recent research by Jonas Frisen at the Karolinska Institute in Stockholm, Sweden has shown that whilst most cortical neurones are 'permanent' (i.e. as old as you are) there is definitely evidence of new neurones being created within the hippocampus of the adult brain. The hippocampus is a small organ located in the brain's medial temporal lobe and forms an important part of the limbic system, the region that regulates emotions. The hippocampus is associated mainly with memory, in particular, long-term memory. The organ also plays an important role in spatial navigation.

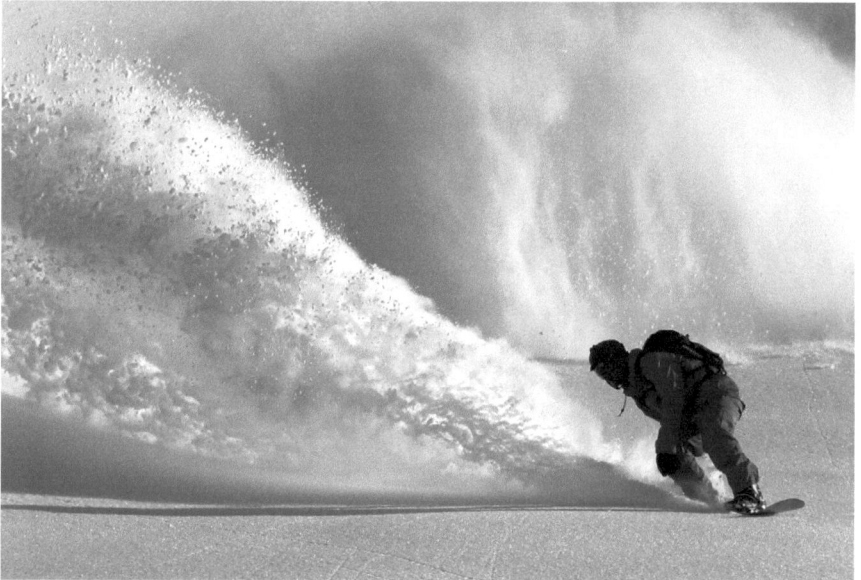

So it is probably a major part of the learning process that we actually create new neurones in this area. Good reason to continually push to learn new stuff at whatever age we may be.

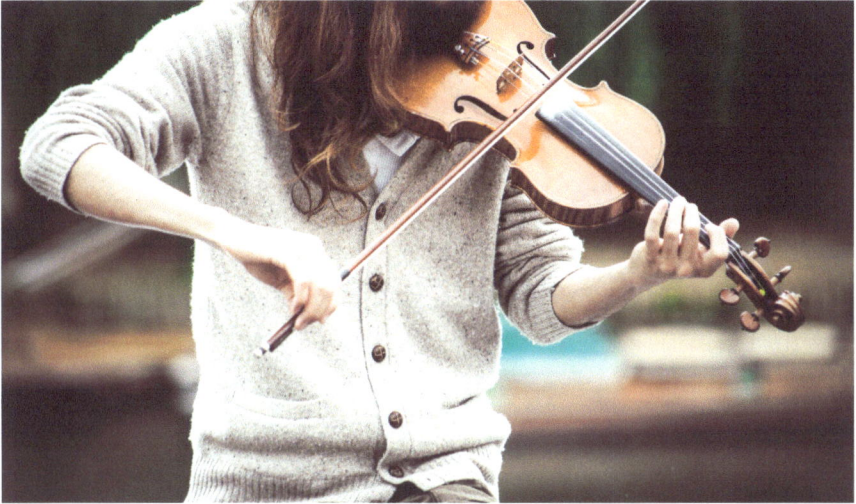

So as the body passes through time some of the organs and tissues degenerate either through some sort of biological clock or through 'wear and tear'. We have known for a very long time some things which may appear to make us age quicker such as sunlight and smoking. We have also known for some time things which appear to make us age slower for example diet and exercise etc. But I think we also need to consider the psychology of the ageing process.

I have said to some of my patients in the past that I don't think I am as old as my father was when he was my age. Whilst this is obviously chronologically inaccurate, what I mean is that my attitude to life seems 'younger' to me than his was. He was a very fit man and even played squash into his early seventies, but I remember him taking us all skiing as a young adult and whilst he did come with us he didn't ski.

He enjoyed watching us have fun and he was obviously capable but somehow felt too old to ski.

Now I may be a little extreme at times but I would certainly be happy to go skiing now. I also took up paramotoring in my late forties and do a whole load of things once seen as the provision of the young.

What I'm trying to get at is I firmly believe that you are only as young or old as you feel. If you think you are too old to do something then you are. If you don't then you aren't. The actual chronological or even biological age is nearly irrelevant. I say nearly as there is some reduction in physical capabilities as we age but even most of that is not inevitable.

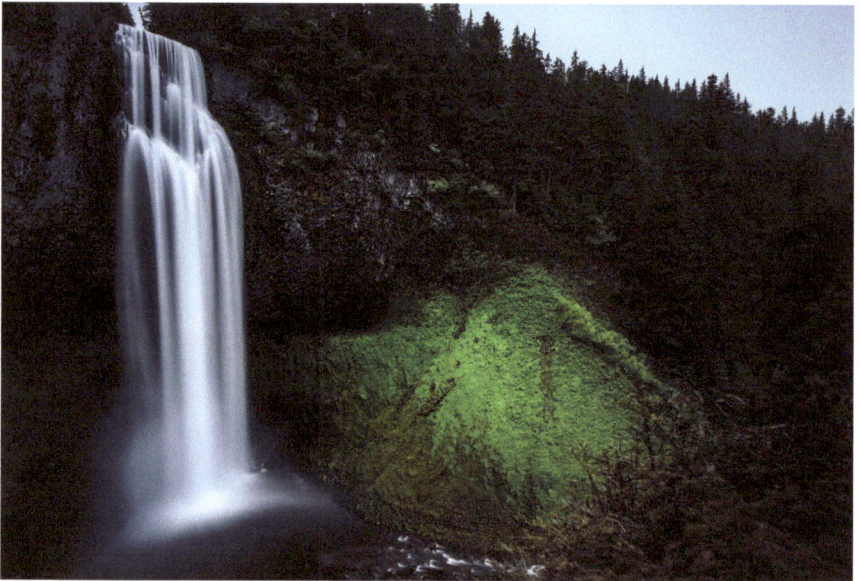

I recently saw a Facebook post about an Indian gentleman who was running the London Marathon at over 90 years of age. Yes, he didn't break any records in his time but he did complete it.

At which point some will say then he must have been doing marathons all his life. No, apparently he did his first marathon at the age of 74. So yes 16 years ago, but his first at 74!

So whilst some physical degeneration is possibly pretty likely I do feel that a lot of the visible deterioration has at least started in the head. People have said to themselves 'I'm too old for that' and thus not even tried.

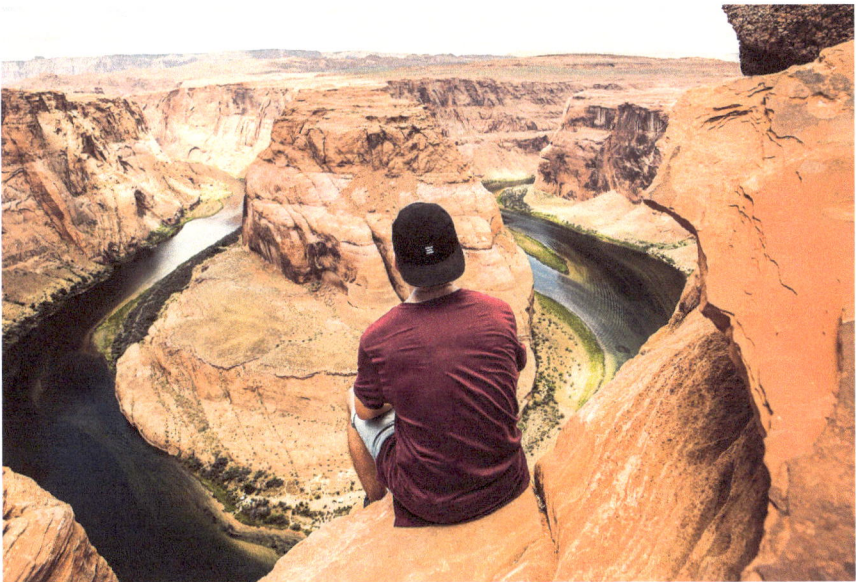

So perhaps the take-home message here is that many of the aspects of ageing that we used to think of as inevitable probably aren't. It certainly seems like a good idea to look after our bodies from a very early age if we intend to keep using them for a long time. Lifestyle, diet, exercise and stress can all shorten our lives at least a bit so let's make choices that will maximise or health and longevity.

I have also frequently said that I have no desire to live to 100 if I spend the last 20 years drooling from the side of my mouth in a hospital bed, but I am quite happy to die at 95 if I was able to go 'white river rafting down the Grand Canyon' at 94.

It is most certainly not about the years in my life but the life in my years.

I'll finish this chapter with a favourite quote.

Life is not measured by the number of breaths we take, but by the number of moments which take your breath away.

Fill your life to the brim with '"wow" moments.

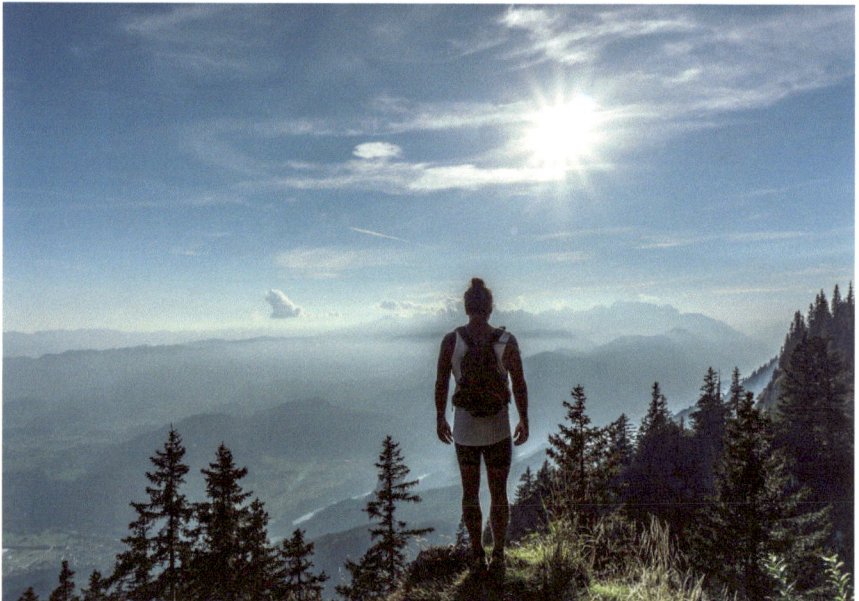

Let me tell you about Telomeres

Ok, some technical stuff here but I'll try to keep it simple. For those who have never heard of them, Telomeres are the DNA equivalent of the plastic tags at the end of your shoe laces.

Each cell of your body contains 23 pairs of chromosomes. Each of these 46 chromosomes is made up of twin strands of DNA tightly coiled around protein structures known as histones. Your genes are coded sequences of this DNA which determine whether you have blond hair or blue eyes etc. The human genome consists of somewhere between 20 and 25 thousand genes. This doesn't sound like very many does it.

There are also areas at the ends of these DNA strands which have been termed 'uncoded'. We originally thought these were functionless but we now believe they may confer some kind of protective function during cellular reproduction. When a cell divides to produce another cell the DNA must be replicated to create another set of chromosomes. This replication is a little less than perfect and some anomalies can creep in. The accumulation of these anomalies might be one of the major reasons for cell senescence and eventual cell death. The telomeres may protect against these anomalies. These uncoded regions at the ends of the DNA start off very long when you are born and gradually get shorter and short-

er as you age. This shortening process is not consistent and some chromosomes will have shorter telomeres than others. So these can be seen to be a marker for cellular age.
We have known for a long time various lifestyle choices which can make this shortening process more rapid and various ones that make it happen more slowly so that all of the things discussed in this book not only make you feel better but may have a direct effect on your telomeres in your DNA.

There are now good and reliable tests that will assess your telomere lengths on a lot of your chromosomes on various cell lines. This can be said to give you a biological assessment of your age, or at least your relative physiological fitness compared to age-matched individuals similar to yourself. This can be a useful and possibly important indicator as to things you might want to change to look after yourself better.

There is also a new area of research looking into products which might stimulate an enzyme in your body called telomerase. This enzyme can possibly lengthen your telomeres and thus 'turn back the clock'.

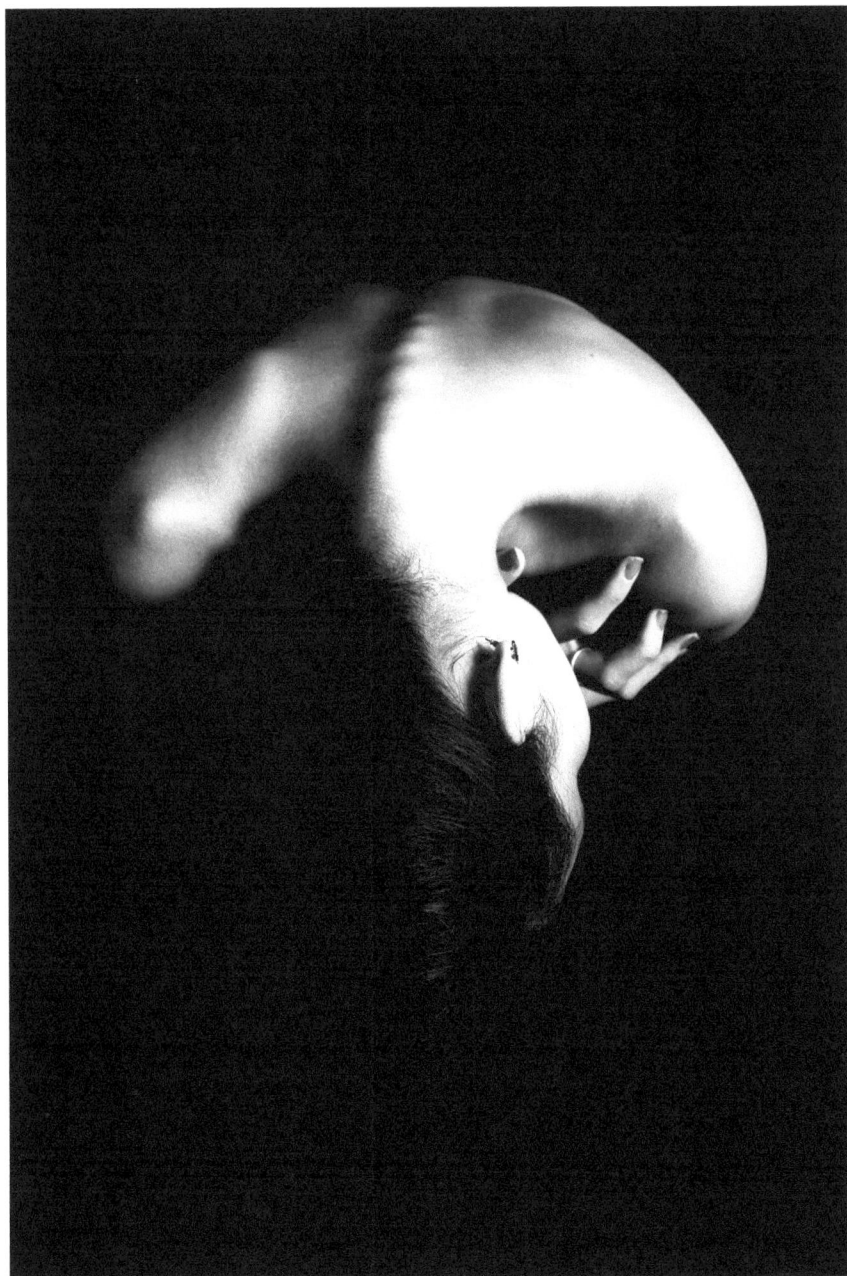

Everyone is an individual

Whilst this next bit might seem a little wishy-washy to some I do think it's crucial. I have tried to write this book in a way that applies to everyone, but nothing does apply to everyone. So this is all designed to stimulate ideas and thoughts and get you to try something new, something different.
Give it enough time and see if it works for you. Make sure you try anything for more than a few days. Changing your life can happen in an instant but making it stick takes practice and perseverance.

We are all individuals and respond differently to the same things. Just because it works for your friend at work doesn't mean it will work for you but it just might. It certainly worth a try.

Also as previously said all diets of any kind produce plateaus. These are periods when you don't appear to be losing any more weight as your biochemistry alters. Don't take these plateaus as a sign that 'this diet obviously doesn't work' (or even 'doesn't work for me'). All you need to do is keep going and your body will adjust and you will start losing again.

The other common finding is that as you approach your ideal weight the weight will start to come off more slowly and that is normal too. So don't let either of these things make you give up.

Why so many different opinions?

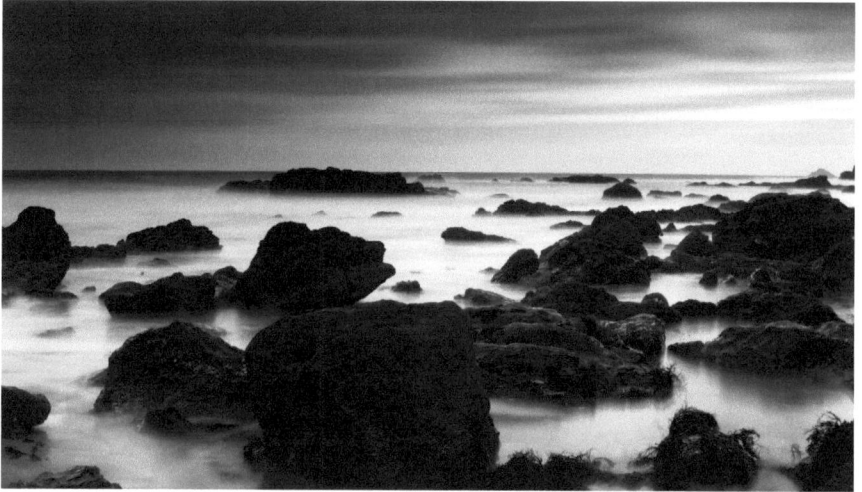

Funnily enough, the last chapter is the main reason why there are so many different opinions. Some people will find something which works for them, which might even contradict what other research has shown may be better and they will promote their own experience over and above the more recent research.

Another reason why there are so many opinions is that medical schools and nutritional training courses often teach from older information and many practitioners stick with advice they have been giving for years regardless of whether any new information had come out which might persuade them to change their tactics.

This is true of many fields but it is particularly true in nutrition.

So despite the very compelling research coming out that suggests the long-running advice for the low-fat diet as being completely wrong there are still plenty of nutritionists and personal trainers and even a fair few doctors who will tell you to stick with the low-fat ideas.

All I can say is please do you own due diligence. The papers are out there. The research is good and compelling and yes we doctors have probably been giving out the wrong advice for over 25 years.

Check it all out and you will see a lot of research backing up what I say.

I have purposely not included links in this text to keep things simple but also to persuade you to do your own research and reading. Looking up a list of references that I have carefully picked out are pretty much bound to agree with me. If you do your own searches you will find the good and the bad, but you will be able to come to a better understanding and decide for yourself who you believe.

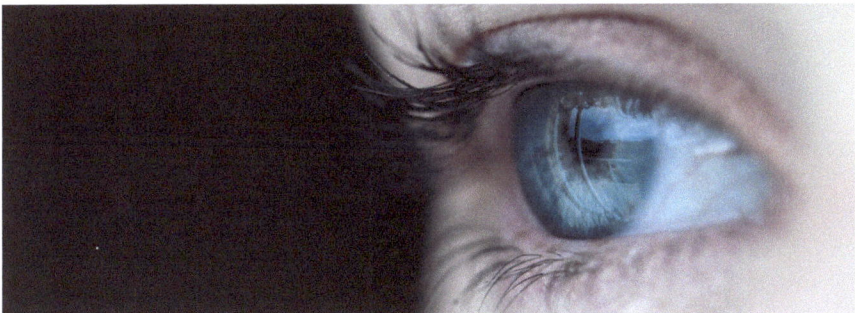

What next?

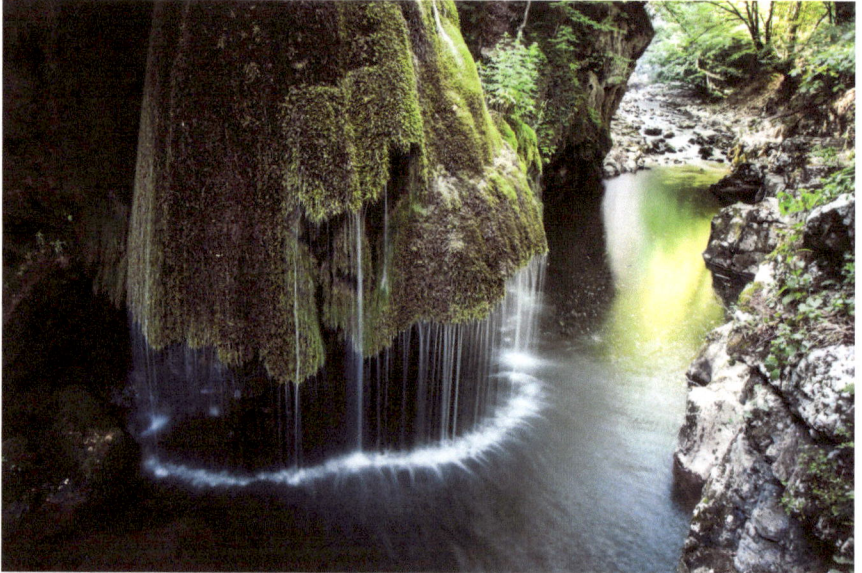

Well, I suppose this is the easy bit. Give it a go. Start small.
Do easy stuff first and as it becomes second nature stretch
yourself to go further.

Let's try to summarise it like this:
Eat real food.
Not too much.
Less starchy stuff.
Skip meals when it's easy.
Move as much as you can.
Put some effort in from time to time.
Don't eat unless you are hungry.

If that is again a bit wishy-washy then try this.

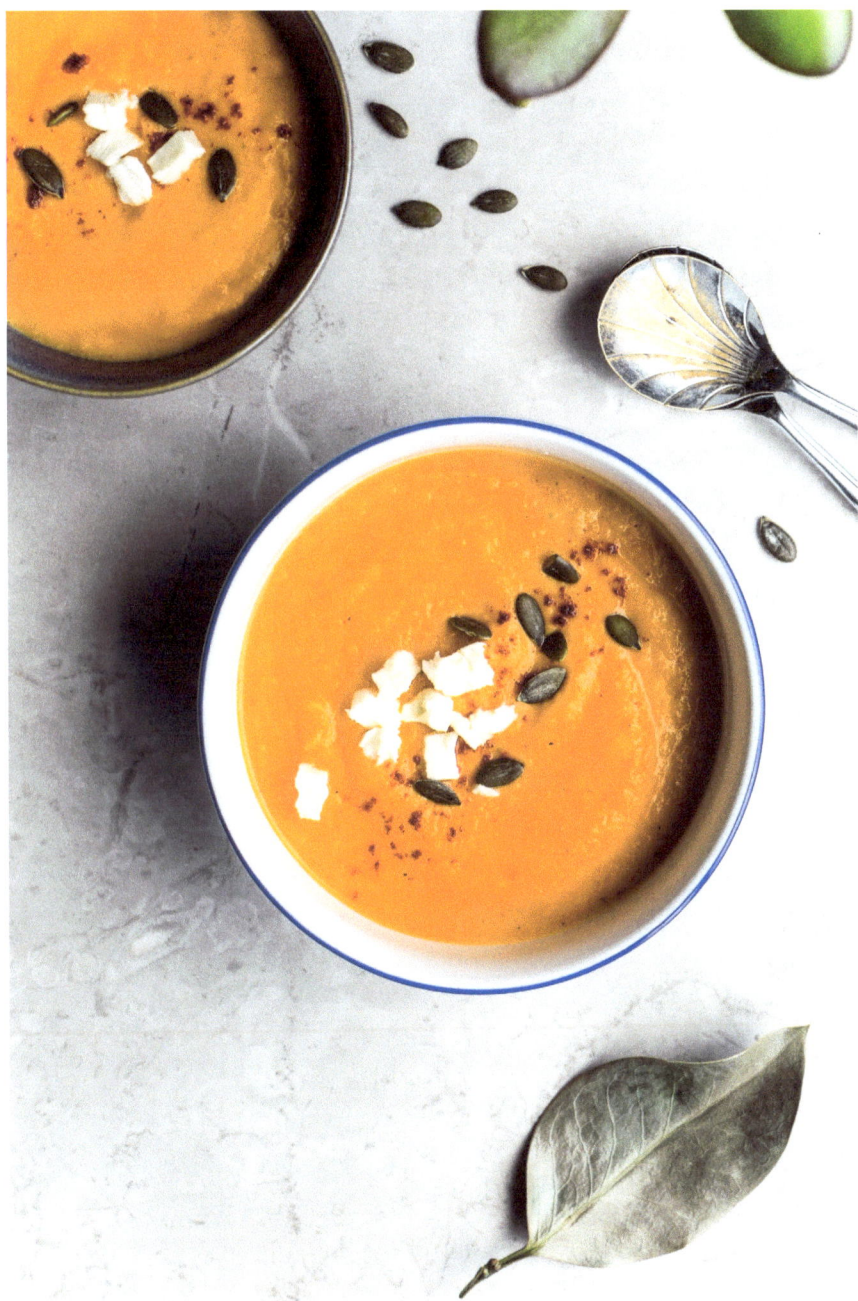

Monday, Wednesday, Friday skip breakfast and lunch then have a light evening meal. Tuesday, Thursday and at the weekend do what you like, don't get stressed about it.

However, and it is a big however, on your feast days don't eat unless you're hungry. Don't eat because it's a particular time of the day. Only eat until you are no longer hungry. Never get full! Full means you ate too much.
Don't treat your mouth as a bin to put the rest of the food in just because you paid for it or it's on your plate.

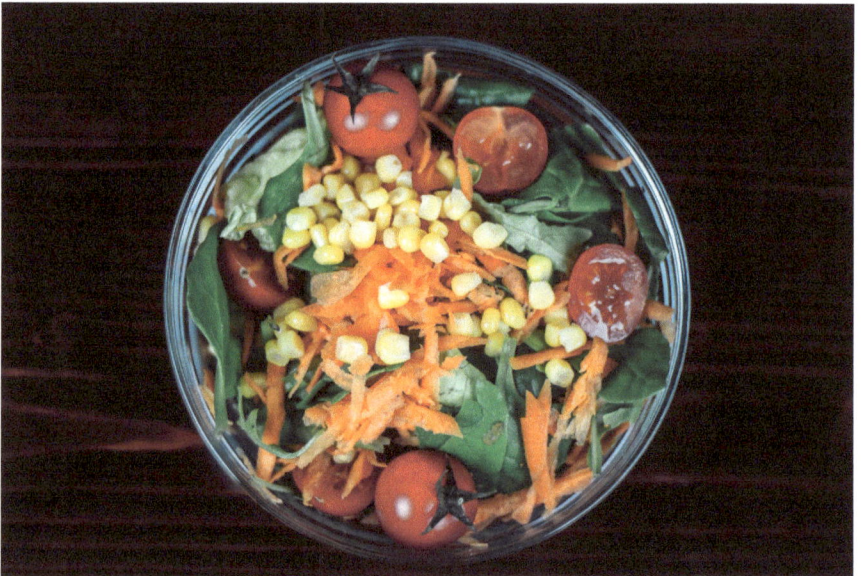

Other than that just relax,
chill out,
smile a bit,
breath.
Life is good.

Finally

I hope you have enjoyed this book. I hope you have learned something new and will give it a go. I hope you are successful in your aims.

I would like to ask you a big favour. If you liked the book and if you found it useful would you please be kind enough to review the book on the Amazon website. They list all validated reviews and these can be very helpful in getting the word out to others who can also benefit from this information.

If you have any questions or comments you would like to address to me feel free to contact me at paulcronin@dr.com.

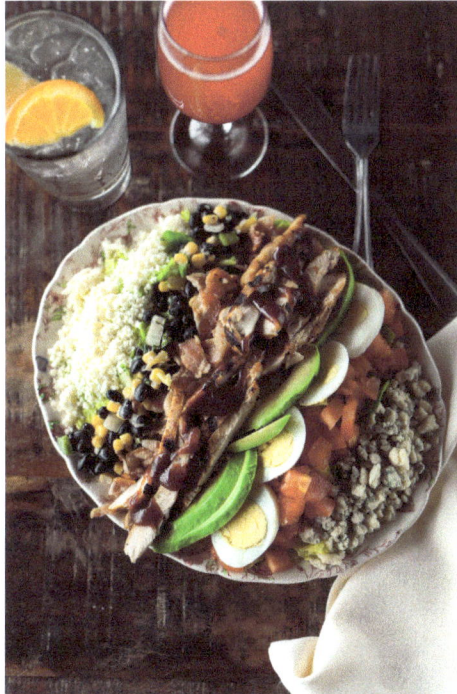

CPSIA information can be obtained
at www.ICGtesting.com
Printed in the USA
BVHW021404210422
634980BV00001B/1